# RACING WEIGHT

*2nd Edition*

# RACING WEIGHT

## *HOW TO GET LEAN FOR PEAK PERFORMANCE*

## MATT FITZGERALD

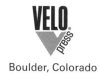

Boulder, Colorado

3002 Sterling Circle, Suite 100
Boulder, Colorado 80301-2338 USA
(303) 440-0601 · Fax (303) 444-6788 · E-mail velopress@competitorgroup.com

Distributed in the United States and Canada by Ingram Publisher Services

Library of Congress Cataloging-in-Publication Data
Fitzgerald, Matt.
Racing weight: how to get lean for peak performance / Matt Fitzgerald.—2nd ed.
    p. cm.
Includes bibliographical references and index.
ISBN 978-1-934030-99-8 (pbk.: alk. paper)
1. Endurance sports—Training. 2. Endurance sports—Physiological aspects.
3. Athletes—Nutrition. 4. Body weight—Regulation. I. Title.
GV749.5.F58  2012
 613.2'024796—dc23

                              2012042138

For information on purchasing VeloPress books, please call (800) 811-4210, ext. 2138,
or visit www.velopress.com.

This paper meets the requirements of ANSI/NISO Z39.48-1992 (Permanence of Paper).

Cover design by Maryl Swick
Cover photograph by Tim Mantoani
Interior design by Vicki Hopewell
Interior photographs on pages 203, 204, 211, 214, 219, 222, 223, 224, and 227 courtesy
    of Corbis; pages 206, 208, 212, 213, 218, and 220 courtesy of Getty Images; page 210
    courtesy of Ray Vidal; page 216 courtesy of Nick Onken; page 226 courtesy of CJ
    Farquharson, CJFoto.com
Illustrations in Chapter 1 and Appendix by Kagan McLeod and Mike Faille

Text set in MillerText

12    13    14 / 10    9    8    7    6    5    4    3    2    1

After the first edition of *Racing Weight* was published in November 2009, I started to receive feedback from athletes who had read it and had implemented the program. It has been gratifying to see the great number of positive results. Most of the athletes who have shared their success stories with me have thanked me for having addressed the long-standing need for a weight-management program designed especially for endurance athletes. I am always quick to point out to these folks that it is *they* who deserve the credit for their results. Yes, I have provided some useful information, but the motivation is theirs, and it makes all the difference.

There are other sorts of feedback that I have received from *Racing Weight* readers as well: questions, points of confusion, a few criticisms, and a correction or two. The book was not perfect. And any program that is based on the best practices of elite athletes and is supported by current science will begin to show its age as best practices evolve and science advances. It's not as if the most successful endurance athletes have started doing anything radically new for weight management or as if the scientific underpinnings of the Racing Weight program have been completely inverted, but over time we reshape these ideas in subtle but important ways.

For example, a colleague of mine, Robert Portman, PhD, who is one of the world's leading sports nutrition researchers, recently made a compelling case in favor of concentrating carbohydrate intake in the early part of the day and protein intake late in the day. A small but growing number of athletes are now practicing this method with good results. Therefore I have chosen to incorporate it into the "nutrient timing" step of the Racing Weight system.

Quite apart from the evolution of athletic best practices and science, my thinking on training, nutrition, and weight management has continued to evolve through my experience as an athlete and coach. Where necessary, I have refined some of the tools presented in *Racing Weight*. The second edition of the book has been a welcome opportunity to address the questions and suggestions of the first edition's readers, to update the program with the latest research, and to make the changes and additions that would make the program even more effective for motivated athletes.

The biggest change is that, whereas the original Racing Weight program comprised five steps, the revised program adds a sixth step: self-monitoring. Research has shown that self-monitoring practices and the

# PREFACE
## TO THE SECOND EDITION

The premise of this book is simple: Weight management is as important for endurance athletes as it is for nonathletes, yet the goal and the best methods of weight management are different for those who race than they are for those who don't.

As a sports nutritionist and journalist I have written a great deal about weight management for both athletes and nonathletes. I must confess that I find it more rewarding to coach athletes toward getting leaner. The secret to weight loss for the overweight nonathlete is motivation. Most people who are really motivated to lose weight are bound to succeed. As they say, "Where there's a will, there's a way." Dieters seldom fail for lack of knowledge. As a weight-management coach of nonathletes, I can only educate; the motivation to succeed has to come from within each individual. If that were easy, obesity wouldn't be so prevalent today.

Endurance athletes are different. The motivation to perform better is intrinsic to members of this group. Cyclists, Nordic skiers, rowers, runners, swimmers, and triathletes are willing to do what it takes to improve, whether it's train harder, take recovery more seriously, work on their mental game—or lose excess body fat.

# CONTENTS

behavioral modifications that surround them are the strongest predictors of successful long-term weight-loss maintenance in the general population. In this regard, endurance athletes are not so different from nonathletes. Readers of the first edition will recall that the book contained a chapter titled "Monitoring Your Progress." However, the monitoring practices described therein were extrinsic to the program. By integrating self-monitoring into the Racing Weight method, you will, I hope, be able to tap this advantage in your effort to reach your racing weight.

Readers familiar with the first edition will notice other changes. I added Chapter 3, "Dieting vs. Performance Weight Management," as a general overview of the Racing Weight program. In it, I explore exactly which weight-management methods athletes can and cannot successfully borrow from nonathletic dieters. Chapter 10, "The Racing Weight Journey," provides additional guidance on how to put into practice the six steps of the Racing Weight program.

Less conspicuous but no less important than these structural changes are some new tools that have been added to the chapters that outline the six steps. These tools are intended to make the program as simple and easy to practice as it can possibly be.

MATT FITZGERALD

# INTRODUCTION

How would your performance change if you were at your optimal body weight? Imagine what it would feel like to set out on a run weighing 10 pounds less than you do right now. How much would it affect your efficiency, your endurance, or, more simply, your self-image? When was the last time you saw a marked improvement in your fitness? Do a few extra pounds stand between you and a faster race? Chances are that it was your quest for optimal body weight that led you to pick up *Racing Weight*.

You are not alone in this quest. Several years ago I assisted exercise scientists from Montana State University in conducting a survey of endurance athletes concerning their attitudes about their body weight and their weight-management practices. More than three thousand cyclists, runners, triathletes, and other endurance athletes responded. Most were serious competitive athletes who trained at least one hour a day, five days a week. The results of the survey, which were presented at a meeting of the Society for Behavioral Medicine in Montreal, Canada and published in the *Annals of Behavioral Medicine* (Ciccolo et al. 2009), were quite interesting.

Seventy-four percent of respondents labeled themselves as "concerned" or "very concerned" about their body weight. Fifty-four percent said that they were dissatisfied with their body weight. These figures are almost identical to those that come from surveys of the general population, despite the fact that the general population is quite a bit heavier than most of the people who took the Montana State survey.

While striking on one level, these findings did not surprise me. That's because, as a sports nutritionist and endurance sports expert, I am accustomed to communicating with and helping endurance athletes who are concerned about and dissatisfied with their body weight. As a runner and triathlete myself, I share their concern and, at times, their dissatisfaction.

The nature of the endurance athlete's concern and dissatisfaction is somewhat different from the nonathlete's, however. The nonathlete is typically motivated to shed excess body fat by a desire to look better and, perhaps also, by a desire to improve his or her health. Endurance athletes care about looking good and being healthy too, but they are equally concerned about their sports performance, and they know that excess body fat is the enemy of performance in every endurance sport. For example, a runner weighing 160 pounds has to muster about 6.5 percent more energy to run the same pace as a runner weighing 150 pounds.

Whereas two-thirds of American adults in the general population are overweight, most of the athletes who took the Montana State survey had body-mass indices that fell within the healthy range. Yet more than half of these endurance athletes reported being heavier than the weight they consider optimal for peak performance in their sport—hence their dissatisfaction. Do these men and women suffer from a distorted body image? By and large, no. They simply have different standards for their bodies, and they struggle to attain them just as nonathletes struggle to meet their own, more relaxed standards. You probably know exactly what I'm talking about.

As much as most athletes appreciate the importance of a lean body composition to endurance performance, I believe that many athletes nevertheless underestimate its impact. They generally assume that while excess body fat may be the greatest performance limiter for athletes who are truly overweight, athletes who are already lean are more likely to be held back by fitness factors such as aerobic capacity. In fact, leanness is as important to performance as any fitness factor at every level of endurance sports, right up to the very top. This was shown in a study involving two dozen elite male and female distance runners from Ethiopia (Beis et al. 2011). All of these runners had very low body fat levels and very fast race times, but the leanest ones had the fastest times. Even though the differences in body fat were small, these differences predicted the variation in their race times as well as differences in aerobic capacity ($VO_2$max).

My own appreciation for the importance of body weight to running performance in particular was heightened by an experience I had in 2008. Darwin Fogt, a Los Angeles–based physical therapist, had invited me to stop by his facility to try out his Alter-G antigravity treadmill. I had been dying to step onto one of these machines since I first heard about them a couple of years earlier, so I readily accepted his offer.

The Alter-G allows the user to walk or run at the equivalent of as little as 20 percent of his or her body weight by increasing the air pressure within an airtight tent that seals around the user's waist and thereby lifts the runner. Many elite runners, including three-time Olympian Dathan Ritzenhein, use it to train through injuries that prevent them from running on their full body weight. Others, such as Ritzenhein's Nike teammate Galen Rupp, use it to increase their running volume without increasing their risk of injury.

A **160** -LB. runner expends **6.5%** MORE ENERGY THAN A **150** -LB. runner at the same pace.

My epiphany came when Fogt zipped me into his Alter-G, increased the belt speed to my normal jogging pace, and then reduced my effective body weight to 90 percent. Instantly I felt as if I had become 10 percent fitter. Scooting along at a 7:00/mile pace was utterly effortless. It was not a feeling of gross artificial assistance, like running on the moon. Rather, it felt like normal running, only so much better.

I was so impressed by the experience that I later used an Alter-G as a tool for helping other athletes to better appreciate the impact of body weight changes on performance capacity. Many of these athletes were shocked by how heavy they felt at their full body weight after experiencing 90 or 80 percent of it. What had felt normal minutes earlier now felt like trying to run while wearing a stuffed backpack. It was a very effective teaching tool that probably motivated more than a few athletes to step up their efforts to get leaner.

Unfortunately, endurance athletes seldom choose the best methods to pursue their optimal racing weight. Despite their awareness of the body weight–performance connection, their hard training, and their efforts to eat carefully, a majority of the athletes in the survey I described said they were currently above their optimal racing weight.

Why do so many endurance athletes struggle to reach and maintain their racing weight? For largely the same reasons that nonathletes struggle to avoid becoming overweight. Our modern lifestyle is different from that of our early ancestors in two important ways that promote excessive weight gain: We have easy access to cheap, high-calorie foods, and we are much less active.

## ENDURANCE ATHLETES SELDOM CHOOSE THE BEST METHODS TO PURSUE THEIR OPTIMAL RACING WEIGHT.

Our early ancestors lived on wild plants, nuts, seeds, and the occasional piece of fish or meat—mostly low-calorie foods and usually just enough of them to supply the energy required to get more food. Today we still have the option to eat like hunter-gatherers, and some nutrition authorities urge people to do so, but it's not a realistic solution for most of us. We have come to prefer the taste of high-calorie foods such as cheeseburgers (which did not exist until a little more than a century ago) to low-calorie foods such as vegetables, and we feel compelled to eat what's put in front of us even though the portions have never been larger and the promotion of food has never been so ubiquitous.

What's more, early humans had to work much harder and burn a lot of calories for every meal, foraging through woods and fields or stalking game for hours, whereas today we just sidle up to a fast-food drive-thru window or press "Start" on the microwave oven. But endurance athletes do have one major advantage over the greater population—we are hardly sedentary. But even most endurance athletes spend more time sitting around than our hunter-gatherer ancestors did, and we are no less plagued by the overabundance of cheap, high-calorie processed foods than our sedentary counterparts.

So if the weight concerns of endurance athletes and nonathletes share a common cause, is their solution also the same? The answer to this question is "yes and no." Certainly, a balanced, natural diet is the most effective means to manage weight for endurance athletes and non-athletes alike. However, the weight management goals of endurance athletes are somewhat different from those of nonathletes, and some of the challenges that endurance athletes face on the path toward an optimal performance weight (rather than toward the basic "healthy body weight" that most nonathletes pursue) are also different. For example, low-carbohydrate diets are an effective weight-loss strategy for nonathletes, but for endurance athletes they are a recipe for disaster because they starve the muscles of the primary fuel they need for endurance performance. Endurance athletes generally require their own special approach to weight management.

Following weight-loss diets that are intended for nonathletes is but one of many mistakes that endurance athletes make in pursuing their optimal racing weight. Relying on supplements, which are marginally helpful at best and dangerous at worst, is another. In 2008, for example, world champion cyclist Marta Bastianelli of Italy was banned from competition after one of her blood samples tested positive for an illegal diet drug. Bastianelli admitted that she had taken the drug after receiving pressure to lose weight from her coaches. More dangerous still is the mistake of disordered eating (usually chronic moderate undereating), which is especially common among collegiate female runners. In a 2007 study nearly one in five female cross-country runners reported past eating disorders and nearly one in four showed evidence of continued inadequate nutrient intake (Thompson 2007). Forcing yourself to go hungry as a means to attain optimal racing weight always backfires in the long run because it deprives your body of the energy needed to absorb hard training.

Not every endurance athlete goes about weight management the wrong way. By definition, the weight-management practices of the highest-performing athletes are the right way to pursue optimal racing weight. This is an important point. The purpose of weight management for the endurance athlete is better performance. The bathroom scale alone cannot determine whether a particular dietary habit or training pattern is effective. The stopwatch is the final arbiter. One of the great things about the competitive nature of endurance sports is that it proves what works and what doesn't. If you want to know the most effective way to train for endurance performance, you can do no better than to study the general training patterns that are shared by the best athletes.

Similarly, if you want to know the right way to manage your weight as an endurance athlete, your best bet is to study the common dietary and weight-management practices of the highest performers.

This isn't a diet book. I wrote this book because I saw a need for a focused, comprehensive, and reliable guide to weight management for endurance sports. It is my belief that such a resource can be truly reliable only if its guidelines are based on the weight-management practices of the best athletes. The Racing Weight system is not some theory of performance weight management that I created by applying creativity to scientific evidence. In this book I've simply presented a description of what works best for endurance athletes in the real world. Furthermore, *Racing Weight* is not dietary shtick that I developed for the sake of having a distinctive brand. My contribution is limited to formalizing this description to some degree by developing tools such as the Diet Quality Score (DQS), which you will learn about in Chapter 4. My work puts me in the happy position of observing what the most successful athletes do, and my service is to pass along what I learn.

There are six specific practices that have stood out to me as the keys to the weight-management success of top athletes and that I believe every other athlete should emulate. Four of them are dietary, one is behavioral, and the last is training related. All six are habits that I have observed over and over again among the most successful athletes in my eighteen years as an endurance sports journalist, coach, and nutritionist. Together these six practices comprise the six steps of the Racing Weight system. Here's a quick synopsis of the plan:

# STEP 1

**IMPROVE YOUR DIET QUALITY.** Step 1 in my Racing Weight plan is improving your diet quality, or the amount of nutrition you get from each calorie in your diet. Increasing the nutrition-per-calorie ratio of your diet will enable you to get all the nutrients you need for maximum performance from fewer total calories, thus enabling you to become leaner. An effective way to improve your diet quality is to grade or score the quality of your current diet and continue to score your diet quality as you make efforts to improve it. Nutrition scientists have come up with various ways of measuring diet quality. Most of these approaches are a bit too complex to be useful to the average endurance athlete, so I created a simplified diet-quality scoring system that you will find very easy to work with and that will help you nourish your body for health and endurance performance. In Chapter 4, I will give you all of the information you need to track and improve your DQS.

# STEP 2

**MANAGE YOUR APPETITE.** It goes without saying that in order to attain and maintain their optimal racing weight, athletes must control the amount of food they eat. But athletes must not go about controlling their food intake by eating less than is required to satisfy their hunger. Not only is this psychologically untenable, but it is also certain to wreak havoc on training performance because physical hunger is closely tied to an athlete's real energy needs. Most athletes, however, eat more than is required to meet their needs and satisfy their hunger. Our modern "food environment" is set up to all but ensure that we overeat without even realizing it.

Fortunately, there are various proven tricks and techniques that you can use to regain control of your appetite and your personal food environment so that you neither overeat nor go hungry. I will share these guidelines with you in Chapter 5.

# STEP 3

**BALANCE YOUR ENERGY SOURCES.** There are three main sources of energy for the human body: carbohydrate, fat, and protein. Many weight-loss diets have been based on the idea that to lose weight, a dieter has to maintain the perfect balance of these three "macronutrients" in daily eating. That none of these diets can agree on the magical macronutrient ratio is not the only evidence that it does not exist.

The best evidence suggests that individuals can balance their energy sources in a variety of different ways with equal success. But for endurance athletes, doing so is a little different because macronutrient balance also has a major impact on training performance and many athletes do not consume enough carbohydrate in particular to maximize that performance. Any measure that boosts your training performance will also tend to make you leaner. In Chapter 6 I will show you how to ensure that you get the right amount of carbohydrate to maximize your training performance and get leaner.

# STEP 4

**MONITOR YOURSELF.** The most common weight-management practices shared by dieters who have lost large amounts of weight and kept the weight off are not dietary patterns such as low fat intake but self-monitoring practices such as weighing and food journaling. Such practices help dieters maintain a high level of awareness of their weight status and a strong commitment to their weight-management goals. Endurance athletes can benefit equally from self-monitoring but need to practice it somewhat differently, monitoring performance as well as diet, weight, and body composition. In Chapter 7 I will present a set of self-monitoring tools designed specifically to help endurance athletes achieve their weight-management goals.

# STEP 5

**TIME YOUR NUTRITION.** When you eat affects your body as much as what you eat. The timing of your food intake has a big impact on what's known as energy partitioning, or what becomes of the calories you consume. There are three main destinations of food calories in your body: muscle, fat cells, and energy. If you want to become leaner, you need to shift the balance of energy partitioning so that more calories are incorporated into your muscles, fewer calories are stored in your fat tissues, and more calories are used to supply your body's immediate and short-term energy needs. This shift will lead to more metabolism-boosting lean tissue and less health-jeopardizing fat tissue.

Interestingly, you can often achieve this objective with little or no reduction in the total number of calories that enter your body. We're really talking about redirecting calories once they've entered your body, not about decreasing the number of calories that enter your body in the first place. The practice of nutrient timing, or consuming the right nutrients at the right times throughout the day, will enable you to partition your energy more effectively and achieve your racing weight. In Chapter 8 I will show you how to practice nutrient timing the way many top endurance athletes do.

# STEP 6

**TRAIN RIGHT.** Despite an increasingly popular belief to the contrary, exercise is the most powerful factor in successful weight management. More than 90 percent of people who succeed in losing large amounts of weight and keeping the weight off exercise regularly. One of the reasons so many people are overweight is that most of them do not exercise regularly.

Endurance athletes by definition have ticked the exercise box of the weight-management checklist. But that doesn't mean that every endurance athlete trains optimally for weight management, and in fact most do not. To begin with, weight management should not be the primary objective of an endurance athlete's training. Performance enhancement should be the primary goal. But these two objectives go hand in hand. If you train optimally to improve your performance, you will also get the best possible weight-management results.

## THE MOST COMMON TRAINING MISTAKE ENDURANCE ATHLETES MAKE IS INSUFFICIENT INTENSITY VARIATION.

By far the most common training mistake in all endurance sports is insufficient intensity variation—specifically a tendency to do almost all training at moderate intensity. However, the best results come from a program in which roughly 80 percent of training is easy, 10 percent is moderate, and 10 percent is hard. In Chapter 9 I will show you how to avoid the most common training mistake as well as other training mistakes, such as insufficient strength training, that limit improvement in performance and body composition.

Part I presents important material that will prepare you to get the most out of the program. In Chapter 1 ("Get Leaner, Go Faster") I will define optimal racing weight in endurance sports generally and in the individual endurance disciplines. In Chapter 2 ("How Much Should You Weigh?") I will help you set a personal racing weight goal. Chapter 3 ("Dieting vs. Performance Weight Management") explains the important differences between the nonathlete's goal of losing weight to look better and be healthier and your goal of attaining your optimal racing weight.

Chapter 4 ("Improving Your Diet Quality"), Chapter 5 ("Managing Your Appetite"), Chapter 6 ("Balancing Your Energy Sources"), Chapter 7 ("Monitoring Yourself"), Chapter 8 ("Nutrient Timing"), and Chapter 9 ("Training for Racing Weight") present the six steps of the Racing Weight system and make up Part II of the book.

Part III provides resources that will help you put the Racing Weight plan into practice. Chapter 10 ("The Racing Weight Journey") ties together the six steps of the Racing Weight program and provides concrete guidelines for implementing the system in the short term and over the long haul. The next chapter, 11 ("Racing Weight Foods"), presents 26 foods that make ideal dietary staples on the Racing Weight plan. Chapter 12 ("What the Pros Eat") presents sample food journals from elite athletes in several different endurance sports. These examples are not to be copied exactly, as there are important differences between the caloric needs of world-class endurance athletes and those of most amateurs, but they do provide some practical ideas and inspiration. In Chapter 13 ("Racing Weight and You") I offer guidelines for special populations such as younger and older endurance athletes.

It takes a certain amount of trust to alter your diet and other lifestyle habits according to another person's advice. My hope is that you find in these pages plenty of reason to put your trust in my program. I am confident that you will, because all of the methods I prescribe are practiced widely by the most successful endurance athletes and are supported by solid scientific evidence. There are also thousands of athletes like you who have already applied the complete Racing Weight system with great results. I know that your trust and commitment will be similarly rewarded. So let's get started!

# FINDING YOUR RACING WEIGHT

## PART I

# ONE

# GET LEANER, GO FASTER

ach sport favors a particular body type. The principle of "form follows function" determines the particular physique that tends to
perform best in a given sport or in a given position or role within
a sport. Certain anthropometric characteristics are advantages
in relation to a sport's specific demands; other characteristics are
liabilities. The most successful basketball players are tall because the
10-foot-high basket favors height. The most successful football lineback-
ers are massive because their job is either to be immovable (offensive
linemen) or to move the immovable (defensive linemen). Tennis players
typically have average builds because their sport requires a combination
of qualities—quickness, power, leverage, balance, and stamina—that
favors no extremes of size or shape.

Endurance sports, of course, tend to favor two related characteristics: low body weight and lean body composition (or a low body-fat level).
This is the case because endurance racing demands the ability to move
economically so that a high work rate (or speed) can be sustained for a
long time and a low body weight and lean body composition contribute
to movement efficiency.

The advantages of being light and lean for endurance performance
are so obvious that they hardly needed to be scientifically proven, but

exercise scientists have gone out and proven them anyway, and the proof is interesting. In a 1986 study Peter Bale and his colleagues at England's Brighton Polytechnic University compared a host of anthropometric measurements in a group of 60 male runners (Bale, Bradbury, and Colley 1986). The subjects were divided into three groups of 20 based on their best 10K race times. The average weight of the men in the "average" group was 152 pounds compared to 145 pounds in the good group and 141 pounds in the elite group. Body composition measurements followed a similar pattern. Average body-fat percentages were 12.1, 10.7, and 8.0 in the average, good, and elite groups, respectively.

## WEIGHT AND BODY-FAT PERCENTAGE ARE MORE STRONGLY CORRELATED WITH FINISH TIMES THAN ARE TRAINING VARIABLES.

It bears noting that even the runners making up the average group were somewhat lighter and significantly leaner than the average nonrunner. The sport selects for naturally lighter and leaner individuals because they generally find greater initial success. The selection pressure continues within the sport right up to the top level. While most world-class runners have similar body weights (with women being lighter than men, naturally), research has shown that within the population of world-class runners, those with the lowest body-fat percentages tend to have the fastest race times.

Studies involving other types of endurance athletes have yielded similar findings. In 2011 Swiss researchers compared anthropometric variables against Ironman® swim, bike, and run split times in a group of 184 age-group triathletes (Knechtle et al. 2011). Body weight was found to have a statistically moderate effect on total race time, while body-fat percentage had a large effect on total race time and a moderate effect (bordering on large) on swim, bike, and run splits. Both body weight and body-fat percentage were more strongly correlated with split times and total race time than are training variables such as average weekly training time.

Interestingly, extra body weight and body fat affected running performance more negatively than swimming or cycling performance in these subjects. The reason is that body weight increases the energy cost of overcoming gravity, and an athlete must overcome gravity with every stride when running but only while going uphill when cycling and not at all when swimming. It's no accident that climbing specialists in cycling are typically lighter than other cyclists. Spanish researchers discovered in a 1999 study that, whereas performance in a flat time trial was best predicted by a rider's maximum power output, performance in an uphill time trial was best predicted by power-weight ratio. The best performers in the uphill time trial tended to be a little less powerful but significantly lighter than the best performers in the flat time trial.

If the major drawback of extra body weight is its effect on the cost of overcoming gravity, then why are the best swimmers and the best cyclists who aren't climbing specialists never very large? There are a few known reasons and probably a few unknown reasons. One is that body weight does also increase the energy cost of cycling on level ground and of swimming.

The amount of energy required to accelerate on a bike is a function of body weight, which gives smaller riders an advantage on criterium courses and other technical courses. Larger riders usually have a larger frontal area as well, making them less aerodynamic. Larger swimmers are less hydrodynamic for much the same reason. While being tall gives a swimmer an advantage of leverage, being broad increases water resistance. This is why the classic swimmer's build is rangy rather than big.

Body weight in the limbs especially increases the energy cost of moving the limbs themselves, reducing what's known as mechanical efficiency. It takes more energy for a cyclist with big legs to turn the pedals and more energy for a swimmer with massive arms to pull and recover.

## ▌■ BODY WEIGHT INCREASES THE ENERGY COST OF OVERCOMING GRAVITY.

Body weight has additional disadvantages that have nothing to do with energy cost. One of the most crucial underpinnings of endurance performance is the ability to deliver oxygen to the working muscles at a high rate. Because large athletes have bigger hearts and lungs and more blood volume, capillaries, and so forth, they are able to consume oxygen at higher rates than smaller athletes, but smaller athletes are able to consume more oxygen relative to their size, which is what really matters. The physiological machinery of oxygen consumption just doesn't scale well to increasing body mass.

It's the same with heat dissipation. The ability to transfer to the environment excess heat generated through muscle contractions is an important performance factor in all forms of long-distance racing. This ability is partly a function of the ratio of body surface area to body volume. This ratio is smaller in bigger athletes, and this is yet another reason that the most successful athletes have low body weights.

The effects of body fat on endurance performance overlap to some degree with those of body weight. Body fat has mass, of course, so the less body fat an athlete has, the less he or she weighs relative to athletes of similar proportions. A certain amount of body fat is required for good health, but any more is just dead weight. Excess muscle is in fact even more detrimental than excess fat because it is far more dense, which is why we're as unlikely to see a muscle-bound Tour de France winner as an obese one. But what constitutes excess muscle is very different from what constitutes excess body fat since muscle is the engine of movement whereas body fat makes no contribution to endurance performance beyond providing energy and even the skinniest runner carries enough body fat to fuel 24 hours of continuous exercise.

## BODY FAT IS A METABOLICALLY ACTIVE ORGAN THAT AFFECTS EXERCISE METABOLISM.

Body fat is far from inert, actually. It is a metabolically active organ that affects exercise metabolism in important ways that are not yet fully understood. One thing we do know is that athletes with larger amounts of body fat burn less fat and more carbohydrate at submaximal exercise intensities. This is not a good thing because the exercise intensity at which the body shifts from burning more fat than carbs to burning more carbs than fat is a strong predictor of endurance performance. If you're an open-water swimmer, for example, the faster you're swimming when you hit this "crossover point," the better you're likely to do in races. Gaining fitness moves this crossover point upward, but losing body fat does too, independent of gains in fitness.

Finally, like excess weight or musculature, excess body fat impedes heat dissipation. It's easier to stay cool on a long ride on a hot summer day if you're very lean. After all, the primary function of body fat is to insulate.

# THE RIGHT BODY FOR THE JOB

While it pays to be light and lean in all endurance sports, there is thankfully no single, ideal body type for any specific endurance sport. The variety you see in the physiques of world-class cyclists, runners, and other endurance athletes can be surprising. For example, the winner of the 1997 Tour de France, Jan Ullrich, stood 6 feet tall and raced at 162 pounds. The winner of the 1998 Tour, Marco Pantani, was 5 inches shorter and more than 30 pounds lighter. Nevertheless, there are certain parameters of body size, proportion, and composition that are characteristic of successful athletes in each endurance sport.

## THE CROSS-COUNTRY SKIER'S BODY

Elite-level cross-country skiers are typically average to slightly above average in height. The average height of male Olympic cross-country skiers is 5 feet 10 inches, and that of their female counterparts is 5 feet 7 inches. Height provides a mechanical advantage for poling, which is important to the generation of forward thrust in cross-country skiing. However, with height comes mass,

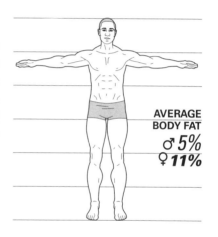

AVERAGE BODY FAT

♂ 5%
♀ 11%

and mass is the enemy of performance in cross-country skiing because it increases gravitational and frictional resistance. That's why you don't see as many 6-foot-5 athletes on the competitive ski trails as you do on, say, the volleyball court.

The typical elite-level cross-country skier is light, but not as light as elites in cycling and running. The average female Olympic cross-country skier weighs 141 pounds, and the average male weighs 165 pounds. The relative heaviness of cross-country skiers compared to some other types of endurance athletes is due to their need for greater upper-body strength, and with strength comes muscle mass. Former U.S. champion Kris Freeman is typically proportioned for an elite male cross-country skier. He stands 5 feet 11 inches and weighs 170 pounds.

While they may be slightly bigger than other endurance athletes, cross-country skiers are among the leanest athletes in any sport. The average male Olympian has just 5 percent body fat and the average female only 11 percent.

## THE CYCLIST'S BODY

There is more than one body type in cycling. The typical physique varies by specialty. Climbers tend to be short of stature and very light. At 5 feet 7 inches and 130 pounds, Marco Pantani was not unusually tiny for a climbing specialist. *Domestiques* and time-trial specialists are typically bigger than climbers. Whereas power-to-weight ratio is the critical variable in climbing, in time trialing it is raw, sustainable

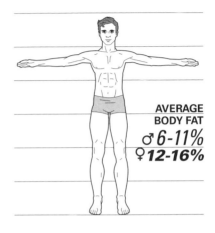

AVERAGE
BODY FAT
♂ *6-11%*
♀ *12-16%*

power output that matters most. Virtually every road-cycling course has some elevation change, though, so it's best not to be too heavy. American David Zabriskie, a seven-time U.S. time-trial champion, has a typical time-trialist build at 6 feet and 147 pounds. Sprinters need to have the ability to sustain high levels of power output over long distances so that they can arrive at the finishing stretch at the head of the peloton, but once there they need the capacity to churn out massive wattage numbers in a short, all-out effort. Sprinters therefore have the most massive legs in cycling and are bigger generally than other cyclists. Sweden's Magnus Backstedt, a Tour de France sprint-stage winner, raced at 210 pounds.

Overall, though, cyclists in all specializations have similar body types. They have twiggy upper bodies like those of runners but with far more muscular legs. Cyclists have greater leg muscularity because the legs do essentially all of the work in cycling, whereas running is a whole-body activity. In addition, the body gets a lot of "free energy" from ground impact in running, whereas in cycling the leg muscles must provide all of the energy for forward motion except when one is riding downhill.

A very low body-fat percentage is another hallmark of successful cyclists. The range of body-fat percentage among male riders in the European peloton is 6 to 11 percent, with an 8 percent average. The range among elite female cyclists is a very low 12 to 16 percent.

The physical demands of cross-country mountain biking (as distinct from downhill mountain bike racing, which is not an endurance sport) are very similar to those of hilly and mountainous courses in road cycling. Thus, the body type of the cross-country mountain biker is the same as that of the climbing specialist in road cycling: very light and lean. Indeed, the top cross-country mountain bikers and the top climbers in road cycling not only have the same bodies but also are sometimes the very same athletes at different points in their careers. The classic case is that of Australian Cadel Evans, who went on to win the 2011 Tour de France on the strength of his climbing after winning a world championship as a mountain biker.

## THE ROWER'S BODY

Rowing is the only endurance sport in which body mass is an actual advantage. Larger rowers have more muscle mass with which to apply force to the oars, which in turn apply force to the water, propelling the boat forward. Of course, more muscle means more power in every endurance sport, but unlike in other endurance sports, that mass comes at no cost in rowing, because there is 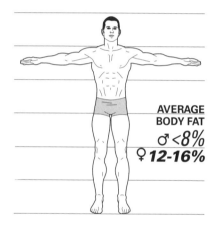 no gravitational resistance to be overcome and the extra body weight has very little effect on frictional resistance between the boat and the water. Indeed, size is such an advantage in rowing that larger rowers and smaller rowers compete in separate divisions.

Steve Redgrave had a typical, male world-class rower's build. At 6 feet 5 inches, and 225 pounds, Redgrave won five rowing gold medals in five Olympics for Great Britain. Anna Cummins is only slightly above average in size for a champion female rower. A member of the U.S. women's eight team that won gold in Beijing, Cummins stands 6 feet tall and weighs 170 pounds.

Yet you won't find any 300-pound elite rowers, and there are three reasons for this. First, rowing is as much a technique sport as it is a pure power sport. Beyond a certain point, muscle mass gets in the way of technique. You could say that you don't see any rowers with arms like bodybuilders for the same reason you don't see any Major League pitchers with such arms. Pitching a baseball is a power action, but it also requires a whiplike arm motion that is inhibited by excess mass. Second, rowing is also an aerobic sport, and many of the muscle characteristics that support aerobic metabolism cancel out those that support muscle growth. Top rowers are born with aerobically powerful muscles, and they further develop aerobic muscle characteristics in training, thus limiting their muscle-mass gains. Finally, rowing training consumes a lot of calories, keeping the athlete's body-fat percentage low, and a human being can become only so heavy with a body composition as lean as that of the typical elite rower.

How lean are top rowers? There is a difference between heavyweight and lightweight rowers in average body-fat percentage. Lightweight rowers tend to be leaner in part because of their special efforts to make weight. Studies have shown average body-fat percentages in the range of 12 to 16 percent for female lightweights and below 8 percent for male lightweights. The averages are slightly higher among heavyweights.

## THE RUNNER'S BODY

Top distance runners are notoriously light and skinny. Former marathon world-record holder Haile Gebrselassie of Ethiopia weighs a scant 117 pounds. Women's 5,000 meters world-record holder Tirunesh Dibaba, also Ethiopian, weighs 97 pounds. And it's all muscle. Exercise physiologists William McArdle, of the City College of New York, and Frank Katch, of the University of Massachusetts (McArdle, Katch,

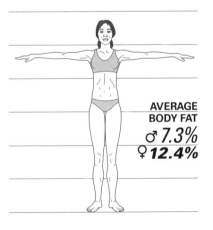

**AVERAGE BODY FAT**
♂ 7.3%
♀ 12.4%

and Katch 2005), among many others, have compiled body-composition data on elite athletes in a wide variety of sports across a number of studies. They found an average body-fat percentage among elite, male marathon runners of just 7.3 percent, which is lower than in any other sport, and an average body-fat percentage among female distance runners of

12.4 percent, which is lower than for every sport except bodybuilding and (of all things) the modern pentathlon.

Body weight is the bane of the distance runner because the runner must move his or her body against gravity—that is, upward—with every stride. A study by researchers at the University of Georgia (Cureton and Sparling 1980) found that a body-weight increase of 5 percent reduced performance by 5 percent in a 12-minute test run.

While you certainly already knew that distance runners are lean and light, you might not have known that elite female runners are average to above average in height (women's marathon world-record holder Paula Radcliffe is 5 feet 8 inches), whereas men are shorter than average. Furthermore, both male and female elites have narrow hips and smaller-than-average feet, and they carry a disproportionate amount of their lower body mass in the upper thighs and less in their lower thighs and shins. All of these features promote running economy.

## THE SWIMMER'S BODY

Swimming is not a natural human activity, so it is no surprise that the typical elite swimmer's body has some unusual characteristics. Successful swimmers are typically tall—often very tall—with unusually long torsos and arms that enable them to slip through the water efficiently and take long strokes. They also have large feet and loose ankles, which add power to the kick. Many elite swimmers

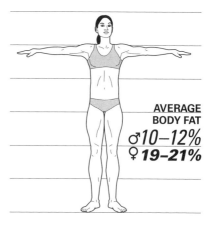

**AVERAGE BODY FAT**
♂ *10–12%*
♀ *19–21%*

are double-jointed in their elbows, knees, and ankles, an anomaly that helps them apply more body-surface area against the water over a greater joint range of motion and thereby produce greater forward impulse.

Swimmers carry more fat than other endurance athletes, although they are still significantly leaner than nonathletes. Fat is more buoyant than muscle, and buoyancy reduces water resistance, so a little extra "insulation" is beneficial to the swimmer as long as it is evenly distributed on the body. The typical male, elite swimmer has 10 to 12 percent body fat, and the typical female has approximately 19 to 21 percent.

An interesting question is whether body-fat percentages are somewhat higher in swimmers than in other endurance athletes because athletes with more body fat tend to excel in swimming, or because swim training does not reduce body-fat levels as much as other aerobic activities, or because swimmers eat more than other endurance athletes. The notion that athletes with more natural fat excel in swimming is contradicted by the many examples of top swimmers, such as Barb Lindquist, who have become triathletes and become leaner. (Lindquist qualified for the 1988 U.S. Olympic Trials in swimming and represented the United States in the 2004 Olympic Triathlon.) But a study by researchers at the University of Florida (White et al. 2005) found that volunteers ate 44 percent more after swimming in cool versus warm water. This finding suggests that the extra layer of insulation that swimmers carry is an adaptive response to frequent exposure to cold water, mediated through the appetite. If so, it's a beautiful example of the body's deep intelligence and how the body naturally changes its form and composition to meet the specific demands placed upon it.

## THE TRIATHLETE'S BODY

As you might expect, the triathlete's body is a hybrid of the swimmer's, cyclist's, and runner's bodies. Pro triathletes tend to be tall, but not as tall as pure swimmers, and there are plenty of shorter triathletes who do quite well. (At 5 feet 4 inches, Australian Greg Welch is one of only two athletes ever to win the ITU Triathlon World Championship, the Duathlon World Championship, and the Ironman World Championship.) Furthermore, the combination of run training and bike training results in legs that are more muscular than those of pure runners and less muscular than those of pure cyclists.

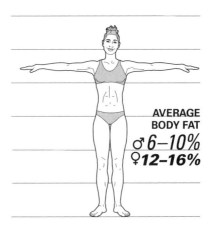

AVERAGE
BODY FAT
♂ *6–10%*
♀ *12–16%*

Interestingly, while most champion triathletes have national-class ability in each of the three triathlon disciplines, virtually none has truly world-class ability in any one of the three. A handful of Olympic-caliber swimmers have crossed over to become dominant triathletes, but nobody that I know of has ever transitioned between the highest level of running or cycling and triathlon, in either direction. Of course, there's Lance Armstrong, who was already a competitive pro triathlete at age 16 (though hampered by a relatively weak run) before he became one of the best cyclists of all time. It seems that past a certain point, the body becomes less suited to the other two disciplines as it becomes better suited to any single one of them. Triathlon demands its own special body type that is distinct from that of the swimmer, cyclist, and runner.

One thing that triathletes do have in common with all other endurance athletes is a lean body composition. Average body-fat levels in male and female pros are 6 to 10 percent and 12 to 16 percent, respectively.

## THE IMPORTANCE OF BEING LEAN

This review of the body types of endurance athletes makes a convincing argument that a low body-fat percentage is the only anthropometric characteristic common to elite athletes in all endurance sports. Not only are top-level athletes quite lean, but also body composition is an excellent predictor of performance at all levels of these sports. For example, in one study (Hecht et al. 2007) researchers found that the average body-fat percentage among age-group (i.e., nonelite) participants in an Ironman triathlon was 17 percent for males and 27 percent for females. These values are lower than average for the general population, but much higher than the values seen in the pros. And sure enough, when the researchers matched body-fat percentages against finishing times, they found that the men and women with the leanest bodies were also the fastest.

Why is a low body-fat percentage so closely associated with better performance in all endurance sports? It's simple. Body fat makes only a minimal positive contribution to endurance performance by providing an energy source. But fat is not the limiting fuel source in any race; carbohydrates are. What's more, any excess body fat beyond the essential level required for basic health worsens endurance performance. Therefore, one of the natural adaptations that the intelligent body makes in response to intensive endurance training is loss of body fat. Specifically, training increases fat metabolism more than it increases appetite. As a result, food intake is insufficient to replace all of the body fat lost during and between workouts, and the athlete becomes leaner. Performance improves as body fat is lost because of gains in efficiency.

The runner has less gravitational resistance to overcome, the swimmer is more hydrodynamic, and so forth. Also, as body-fat levels go down, aerobic capacity goes up, because muscle has less competition from fat tissue for oxygen and fuel. Excess body fat is also known to increase thermoregulatory strain during exercise, so by shedding fat, athletes can go faster without overheating. Endurance athletes who are genetically lean and who become leaner more readily in response to training tend to perform better than their competitors who are not so genetically blessed.

## WHAT YOU CAN DO

You cannot change your height, the width of your hips, the length of your feet, or any of several other anthropometric variables affecting endurance performance that I have discussed in this chapter. You can't change your genetic potential for leanness, either. But you can reduce your body-fat percentage (and thereby adjust your weight) to the level that is optimal for performance in your chosen endurance sport given your unchangeable genetic constraints.

If endurance training automatically pushes body composition toward the optimal level of leanness, and if you are not just beginning as an endurance athlete, then why haven't you reached your optimal racing weight and body-fat percentage already? The answer, as I suggested in the Introduction, is that the modern lifestyle, with its high-calorie processed foods and all-day sitting, tends to counteract the effects of training. In addition, certain common training errors keep many athletes above their optimal racing weight and limit their performance.

In effect, your training and the rest of your lifestyle are sending your body mixed messages. Errors aside, your training is telling your body, "Let's get leaner," while at the same time your diet (or certain features of your diet) and your inactivity outside of workouts are telling your body, "Let's fatten up!" Your body is very intelligent, and it is perfectly capable of "getting the message" and becoming a lean, mean racing machine if you are willing to bring your overall lifestyle into line with that goal. In Part II we will begin to do just that. First, however, let's determine your optimal racing weight, set an initial racing weight goal, and establish a mind-set for long-term success—measures that in themselves will help you get leaner by enhancing your focus, awareness, and motivation.

# TWO

# HOW MUCH SHOULD YOU WEIGH?

magine yourself devoting the next few months to getting in great shape. You train consistently and progressively, pushing hard enough to reach beyond previous limits, yet remaining cautious enough to avoid injuries and overtraining. Your diet is managed with equal care. You load up on wholesome foods and keep indulgences to a minimum, providing your body with abundant fuel and raw materials for repair and maintenance but without excess. The whole process culminates in a big race in which you achieve a breakthrough performance.

If you weighed yourself on the day of this race, the scale would almost certainly display a different number than your current weight—probably a smaller number. This number represents your *optimal performance weight*—that is, the weight that is associated with your highest athletic performance level. (In reality, it may take you longer than one training cycle—a period of training typically lasting 12 to 24 weeks and culminating in a peak race—to reach your optimal performance weight. But for the purposes of this example, let's assume that you are within one training cycle of your optimal performance weight.)

As we saw in the previous chapter, body weight affects performance in every endurance sport. Therefore, as you train and fuel your body toward peak performance, your body adjusts its mass (and composition) to accommodate the demands you're making on it. This change is as significant as any other of the many adaptations that your body makes to accommodate your demand for higher performance, including growth of the heart muscle, greater blood vessel elasticity, and increased muscle glycogen fuel storage.

The process is not as straightforward as simple weight loss, however. Suppose that after your big race you allow yourself to get out of shape and gain some weight. A couple of months pass, and—predictably enough—you begin to grow weary of feeling soft and slow, and remembering your optimal performance weight, you set a goal to reclaim it. Except this time, in your haste, you try to get there more quickly by dieting—that is, by sharply cutting your food intake. It seems to work—on one level, anyway. Before long, the scale displays the same reading it did on the day of your last big race. But there's a problem: You're not nearly as fit. That's because you've undernourished your body and consequently lost a lot of muscle along with some fat. So while your body weight is the same as it was when you were in peak shape, your body composition is different—you have a higher body-fat percentage.

You see, when you're in peak shape, you are not only at your optimal body *weight*; you're also at your optimal body *composition*. It's important to consider both of these factors, because you can be at your optimal body weight without being at your optimal body composition and vice versa. From here on, then, I will use the single term "optimal performance weight" (and, alternatively and more casually, "racing weight") to refer to the combination of optimal body weight and optimal body composition.

There is no simple formula for determining your optimal performance weight. Most endurance athletes calculate it by working to achieve peak fitness and then measuring their weight and body composition at that time. But what is peak fitness? Even when you've just had the best race of your life, how do you know you can't perform even better in the next training cycle? Your highest performance level is fundamentally unknowable, except in retrospect, and so, therefore, is your optimal performance weight. Even so, most endurance athletes know when they are close to the highest performance level they are capable of achieving in their sport. And by definition, if you're close to your ultimate performance level, you're close to your optimal performance weight. So although optimal performance weight cannot be determined with perfect certainty, it can be quantified within a small margin of error.

It is still useful to estimate your racing weight because it allows you to pursue your optimal performance weight as a semi-independent goal. Having such a target will encourage you to fine-tune your training and nutrition in ways that optimize your weight and body composition faster and enhance the performance benefits that you get from approaching your optimal performance weight.

Creating an advance estimate of your optimal performance weight is also helpful for those who feel that they are not as lean as they should be even when they are in peak shape. There are plenty of endurance athletes whose performance is held back by an apparent inability to reach their optimal performance weight. Obviously, these people cannot determine their optimal performance weight simply by stepping on a body-fat scale on the day of a big race. The problem is not that the definition of optimal performance weight as an athlete's body weight and composition at peak fitness fails to apply to everybody. The problem is that an apparent inability to reach optimal performance weight prevents some athletes from achieving peak fitness.

In this chapter I will show you a simple, step-by-step process that you can use to determine your optimal performance weight through the actual training process. I will also show you a unique method of estimating your optimal performance weight before you achieve it. Although this estimate is almost certain to be slightly too high or too low, it will increase the likelihood that you eventually will reach your optimal performance weight, whatever it turns out to be. But before we get into all of that, let me warn you against thinking of the number you identify by the end of this chapter as a *definitive* calculation of your optimal performance weight.

## THE TROUBLE WITH FORMULAS

Most adults have some sense of how much they should weigh. If you picked a man or woman on the street at random and you asked this person to name his or her ideal body weight (don't ever try this experiment!), this person would most likely be able to give you an exact number without hesitation.

Where do such numbers come from? I'll tell you where they don't come from: They don't come from the body-weight tables and formulas created by health experts. These tables and formulas, which include height-weight charts used by life insurance companies and body-mass index guidelines used widely by doctors, are far too general to help individual men and women determine an *ideal* body weight. Their main purpose is to quantify the relationships between body size and health throughout the population so that life insurance companies can better judge the risk of insuring their customers and so that doctors have a statistical basis for advising their overweight patients to slim down. Consider the specific example of body mass index (BMI), which is your weight in kilograms (1 kg = 2.2 lbs.) divided by the square of your height in meters (1 m = 3.28 ft.). All of the possible BMI values are lumped into just four classifications, which are based on health risks:

| BMI | CLASSIFICATION |
| --- | --- |
| Below 18.5 | Underweight |
| 18.5–24.9 | Normal |
| 25–29.9 | Overweight |
| Above 30 | Obese |

These broad classifications are not really helpful in determining ideal body weight for most individual men and women—where "ideal weight" could reflect optimal health or the weight at which you look your very best. For example, a person who stands 5 feet 5 inches tall is considered to be of "normal weight" whether he or she weighs 150 pounds (at 24.96 BMI) or 114 pounds (at 19.0 BMI). Presumably, at that height, your healthiest and sexiest body weight is somewhere in that 36-pound range—but where exactly?

Medical science can't say. First of all, there is no single body weight that is optimal for every person of any given height (I'll explain why momentarily). Nor does medicine have metrics that would enable doctors to pinpoint any single person's optimal body weight. The medical definition of optimal body weight, if it existed, would certainly be the weight at which a person's body functions best. But how do we define functioning best? Theoretically, tests of heart disease risk factors, insulin sensitivity, kidney function, aerobic capacity, sleep quality, and so forth could be used to triangulate this number with some degree of precision, but now we're in the realm of experimentation. In other words, this method could not work prescriptively. It could not identify your optimal body weight until you had already achieved it.

So, then, if we cannot determine ideal body weight using BMI charts and height-weight tables, how does the average person determine his or her ideal body weight? One factor is past experience. Many men and women who are not satisfied with their current weight can look back to a time when they were more satisfied, and they yearn to weigh what they weighed then. The mirror is another important factor. Most people have a sense of how they would like to look, and by looking in the mirror and mentally subtracting the excess body fat they see, they can estimate how much weight they would have to lose to look that way. You are probably getting closer to identifying that number already.

Nobody knows our bodies better than we do ourselves, so there's no reason to doubt the general validity of such methods of determining an ideal body weight. However, they are not perfect. In our society, on the one hand, all too many people, women especially, develop an unhealthy you-can't-be-too-thin mentality that causes them to chase an unrealistically low body weight. On the other hand, there is evidence that as people become heavier and heavier, their perceived ideal body weight also inflates. In other words, while there are more people today who wish they were lighter than they are, as a population we no longer dream of being as light as we used to dream of being. If the average person 20 years ago weighed 160 pounds and wanted to weigh 150 pounds (this is a gross oversimplification for the sake of illustration), then the average person today weighs 175 pounds and wants to weigh 160 pounds. Whereas in the past people wanted to attain what was perhaps a closer-to-true ideal weight, today most people simply want to be not quite so heavy while still believing they want to attain their ideal weight.

Athletes are in a similar predicament to that of the general population with respect to weight. There is no formula that can tell you as an endurance athlete what your optimal performance weight is. While we do have information about the weight and body composition of elite athletes in the various endurance sports, this information cannot serve as a tool to help other endurance athletes in the same sport determine their own optimal performance weight. After all, weight and body composition are determined largely by our genes. A Wake Forest University study (Hsu et al. 2005) found that body-fat percentage is 64 percent inherited.

Lean parents tend to have lean children and fat parents tend to have fat children, regardless of differences in lifestyle. This means that if your parents carry a lot of excess body fat, it is unlikely that you can ever become as lean as the top athletes in your sport, most of whose parents are also naturally lean.

It is not necessarily impossible, though. Lifestyle still controls roughly 36 percent of your body-fat percentage, and it even affects the very genes that regulate your body composition. Finnish researchers (Mustelin et al. 2008) recently compared "discordant" identical twins (one obese, one not obese) and "concordant" identical twins (both nonobese) and found that, even though both twins in the pairs with one obese member were more likely to have certain genes that slowed metabolism, making them predisposed to obesity, these genes were significantly less active in the nonobese member of the discordant pairs, who tended to have a much higher fitness level. These results suggest that exercise switches off some of the genes that work to make you fat—almost as though you had not inherited these genes in the first place.

**BODY FAT IS**

**64%**

**GENETIC &**

**36%**

**LIFESTYLE**

Another factor that makes optimal performance weight nearly impossible to estimate is the long-term influence of your lifestyle, body weight, and body composition throughout your life. As most of us know from experience, body fat is easier to put on than to take off. This is because storing excess fat on your body is different from other forms of storage, such as dumping grain into a silo. After all, dumping grain into a silo does not change the silo. But the fat that you add to your body during periods of weight gain affects your whole body in lasting ways that make this fat resistant to subsequent breakdown. Your insulin sensitivity decreases, making it harder to build and fuel muscle tissue and easier to store even more body fat. Your appetite adjusts to support a higher body weight. And if you reduce your eating despite your increased appetite, your resting metabolism slows down, at least temporarily, to conserve those fat stores, much as you might switch to driving a smaller car to conserve gas in response to rising fuel prices. In sum, gaining fat alters your body's "set point" for weight and composition so that after a period of significant weight gain, it may no longer be realistic to pursue levels of lightness and leanness that might have been realistic before.

There is some evidence that fat stored above the body's midline is broken down more easily than fat stored below the waist. Therefore, so-called apple-shaped individuals may lose their excess body fat more easily than so-called pear-shaped individuals. Unfortunately, women are more likely than men to be pear-shaped, and studies show that overweight men generally lose weight faster than equivalently overweight women on the same weight-loss program. But there are plenty of men and women who are able to become very lean even after gaining large amounts of excess fat in their hips and thighs. The bottom line is that you just never know what's possible for you until you have trained and fueled your way into peak form.

## TIPPING THE SCALES IN FAVOR OF PERFORMANCE

Some athletes have it easy. They are naturally very lean and have always been active, so their weight and body composition don't change much as they pursue the perfect race. Even when they take time off from training or let their dietary standards slip somewhat for a short period of time, there is little change in their physical form. These fortunate athletes discover their optimal racing weight very quickly and are never uncertain about it.

Most endurance athletes do not have it so easy. Their weight and body-fat levels are sensitive to changes in their diet and training. When they don't eat right or train consistently, they put on fat; when they eat better and get on a roll in their training, they lose fat. As they begin their pursuit of the perfect race, these athletes carry substantial excess fat that they need to lose, and it may take them some time to discover their optimal racing weight. It may take even longer if they pursue their optimal racing weight in some of the wrong ways, such as undereating.

Australian triathlete Chris McCormack (known as Macca) is a great example of how the journey toward discovering ideal racing weight unfolds for athletes who are not naturally in the 99th percentile of leanness. Macca is a naturally big man. He's just shy of 6 feet tall and settles into a weight of 185 pounds during periods of lighter training. McCormack was already an accomplished short-course triathlete when he decided to step up to the Ironman World Championship in Hawaii in 2002.

Aware of the notorious heat in Kona, and understanding that larger athletes have a much harder time staying cool when racing in hot environments, McCormack decided he needed to get as light as he possibly could by any means necessary. This was a mistake. Macca failed to finish his first Ironman. Slow to learn the right lesson, he struggled the next few years as well. Today it all seems so clear: "I have definitely gone to the far extreme of being way too light for my body structure," McCormack told me in an interview for *Triathlete*. "My first few years in Kona I was petrified of the heat and was racing at 171 pounds. I would starve myself to get my weight down to the realms I thought were necessary for a bigger guy to deal with the heat."

After another disappointing finish in the 2006 Ironman, McCormack had an idea. That year an uncharacteristically weak bike leg was to blame for his lackluster sixth-place finish. Normally one of the sport's strongest cyclists, Macca was outsplit by 25 other competitors on the bike. He realized that his efforts to get as light as possible had weakened his legs and reduced his cycling ability.

"I just had to find a way to get as light as I possibly could without losing my strength and then build a racing plan that suited the conditions and my issues in them," he told me.

In 2007 McCormack arrived on the Ironman starting line weighing 177 pounds—more than he had weighed in his five previous trips to Kona. And for the first time in six total attempts he won the race, becoming the heaviest Ironman winner ever.

In the following years Macca continued to fine-tune his weight and body composition through subtle changes in his diet and training. This wasn't a matter of trying to fix what was no longer broken but of understanding that there are always ways to improve. When McCormack won his second Ironman World Championship title in 2010, he did so at 175 pounds—a little lighter and, according to him, measurably leaner in the core than he had been when winning his first title, thanks to an increased focus on speed development.

You might assume that Chris McCormack was frustrated by his struggle to find his optimal racing weight for Ironman, but he wasn't as discouraged as you might think.

"I really enjoy the game of managing weight and speed and monitoring my body's feel at different weights," he said.

This great attitude is one that every endurance athlete should emulate. The *only* way to determine your optimal racing weight is to discover it through experience, and the *only* way to attain your optimal racing weight is to focus on performance. If you eat and train for maximum performance, you will ultimately achieve your best performance, and your weight and body-fat percentage on that day will define your optimal racing weight. In the meantime, be patient and enjoy the mental challenge of trying to figure it all out.

> THE ONLY WAY TO ATTAIN YOUR OPTIMAL RACING WEIGHT IS TO FOCUS ON PERFORMANCE.

To determine your optimal racing weight through performance, you must continually monitor your performance alongside changes in your body weight and body composition. I'll show you how to do that in Chapter 7.

## ESTIMATING YOUR RACING WEIGHT

You may find it helpful to estimate your optimal performance weight before you discover it experientially. Many athletes train hard and eat right (or so they think) and yet still have a visible excess of flab on their tummies, hips, and/or thighs even when they are in race shape. If you are at just such an impasse, you may find it helpful to estimate how much more fat you can reasonably expect to lose with further refinements to your training and diet. This estimate might not be completely precise, but it can give you a goal and a target that will encourage you to modify your training and diet in new ways to make you leaner, lighter, and faster.

For that matter, generating an estimated optimal performance weight can be helpful to any endurance athlete who has not yet gone through the process of determining it functionally. After all, working your way into peak shape takes many weeks. And since you're reading this book on racing weight *now,* you would probably like to know now at least approximately what your racing weight should be so that you can go after it consciously the same way you consciously go after race performance goals. Numbers are powerful motivators. In all domains of human endeavor, we typically achieve more when we quantify our goals than we do when we just go by feel. For this reason, I encourage all endurance athletes to estimate their optimal performance weight even before they have a chance to determine it functionally, even though there is no absolutely reliable way to create such an estimate. What the optimal performance weight estimation method I'm about to show you lacks in accuracy it makes up for in practical benefit. It makes you more conscious of the effects of body weight and composition on your performance, more aware of the training methods and dietary habits that affect your weight and fat levels, and more focused on and motivated to achieve your optimal performance weight. Once you have achieved it, you can do away with estimates and use the numbers you arrived at functionally to give you the same benefits in the future.

Generating an estimate of optimal performance weight (which, remember, includes a body-weight number and a body-fat percentage number) really amounts to setting an initial performance weight goal. This method is designed to generate realistic goals, but you're just as likely to exceed the target as to fall short of it. Either way you will end up with a lean body that is fit for maximum performance.

**STEP 1** **FIND YOUR BODY-FAT PERCENTAGE.** To generate an estimate of your optimal performance weight, you will need to get an initial body-fat measurement. The easiest and most affordable way to measure your body-fat percentage (but not the most accurate) is to step on a body-fat scale, but there are other methods. I will briefly discuss all of them in Chapter 7.

After you conduct an initial body-fat test, go to Table 2.1 and find the column for your gender and age group. Then find the percentile that most closely corresponds to your result. For example, suppose you are a 40-year-old woman and your initial body-fat measurement is 26.5 percent. The closest match in your table is 26.4 percent, which corresponds to the 50th percentile for your gender and age group. This means your body-fat percentage is lower than that of exactly half the people in your gender and age group.

Table 2.1 is based on data collected from thousands of body-fat tests performed on men and women of all ages. These data have been used to create percentile rankings for men and women in various age brackets, and they can show how you compare against a broad population that is skewed toward the athletic. The numbers in Table 2.1 are significantly lower than those in the general population (as we saw earlier in the chapter), because the data come from a self-selected group, and those who volunteer for body-fat testing tend to be much leaner than those who do not. But, of course, this very fact makes the numbers more relevant to athletes like you.

**STEP 2** **ESTIMATE YOUR OPTIMAL BODY-FAT PERCENTAGE.** Once you find your current body-fat percentage, use Table 2.1 to define your goal. Most endurance athletes, including beginners, are genetically capable of reaching at least the 80th percentile for their gender and age group. In other words, most endurance athletes can sculpt a body that is leaner than those of 8 out of 10 persons in their reference group. If your current body-fat percentage is between the 40th and 70th percentiles for your age and gender group, an initial goal of reaching the 80th percentile is reasonable. For example, if you are a 52-year-old male and your current body-fat percentage is 21.5, placing you in the 60th percentile for men aged 50 to 59, then set a goal of lowering your body-fat percentage to 17.9, which is defined as the 80th percentile for your group.

In setting your body-fat percentage goal, you can "split the difference" when your current body-fat percentage places you between rows of Table 2.1. For example, if you're a 35-year-old male whose current body-fat percentage is 14.4, you're almost exactly between the 75th percentile (14.9 percent) and the 80th percentile (13.9 percent) for your reference group. The appropriate goal for you is to move up two rows in your column on Table 2.1. To make your goal more accurate, go ahead and set a target to reach a body-fat percentage that is roughly halfway between the body-fat percentage associated with the 85th percentile (12.7) and the body-fat percentage associated with the 90th percentile (11.3). A target of 12.0 percent would be about right in this case.

Let's look at an example of estimating optimal body weight. Suppose your current body weight is 170 pounds, your current body-fat percentage is 14.4, and, as a 35-year-old male, your body-fat percentage goal is 12.0 percent (moving you two rows up from halfway between the 75th and 80th percentiles to halfway between the 85th and 90th percentiles).

To determine how many pounds of body weight you will lose in lowering your body-fat percentage from 14.4 to 12.0, first calculate your current lean body mass. This is the portion of your body weight that consists of stuff other than fat (muscle, bone, etc.), and it won't change much as you shed body fat to get leaner. Since your current body-fat percentage is 14.4, you know that the other 85.6 percent of your current body weight consists of lean body mass. Multiplying your current body weight by your current lean body mass percentage yields your current lean body mass: 170 lbs. × 85.6 = 145.5 lbs.

### TABLE 2.1 BODY-FAT PERCENT POPULATION PROFILES

Locate the body-fat percentage closest to your own current number.

| GOAL | PERCENTILE | MEN 20–29 | 30–39 | 40–49 | 50–59 | 60+ |
|---|---|---|---|---|---|---|
| | 99 | 2.4 | 5.2 | 6.6 | 8.8 | 7.7 |
| | 95 | 5.2 | 9.1 | 11.4 | 12.9 | 13.1 |
| | 90 | 7.1 | 11.3 | 13.6 | 15.3 | 16.3 |
| | 85 | 8.3 | 12.7 | 15.1 | 16.9 | 17.2 |
| IMPROVE 10% | 80 | 9.4 | 13.9 | 16.3 | 17.9 | 18.4 |
| | 75 | 10.6 | 14.9 | 17.3 | 19.0 | 19.8 |
| | 70 | 11.8 | 15.9 | 18.1 | 19.8 | 20.3 |
| | 65 | 12.9 | 16.6 | 18.8 | 20.6 | 21.1 |
| IMPROVE TO 80% | 60 | 14.1 | 17.5 | 19.6 | 21.3 | 22.0 |
| | 55 | 15.0 | 18.2 | 20.3 | 22.1 | 22.6 |
| | 50 | 15.9 | 19.0 | 21.1 | 22.7 | 23.5 |
| | 45 | 16.8 | 19.7 | 21.8 | 23.4 | 24.3 |
| | 40 | 17.4 | 20.5 | 22.5 | 24.1 | 25.0 |
| | 35 | 18.3 | 21.4 | 23.3 | 24.9 | 25.9 |
| | 30 | 19.5 | 22.3 | 24.1 | 25.7 | 26.7 |
| | 25 | 20.7 | 23.2 | 25.0 | 26.6 | 27.6 |
| IMPROVE 25% | 20 | 22.4 | 24.2 | 26.1 | 27.5 | 28.5 |
| | 15 | 23.9 | 25.5 | 27.3 | 28.8 | 29.7 |
| | 10 | 25.9 | 27.3 | 28.9 | 30.3 | 31.2 |
| | 5 | 29.1 | 29.9 | 31.5 | 32.4 | 33.4 |
| | 1 | 36.4 | 35.6 | 37.4 | 38.1 | 41.3 |

*Source:* Compiled from data collected by Kip Russo, founder of Body Fat Test, Inc.; reproduced with permission. Russo used a testing method called hydrodensitometry, one of the most accurate methods of body-fat measurement.

**STEP 3** **CALCULATE YOUR OPTIMAL BODY-WEIGHT TARGET.** You will use your optimal body-fat percentage to do this. When you reach your optimal body-fat percentage of 12.0, your lean body mass will remain approximately 145.5 pounds, because you will not lose any muscle or bone, only fat. But your lean body mass will now account for 88 percent of your total body weight instead of only 85.5 percent. Representing your new body weight as $X$, use the following equation to calculate its value: 145.5 lbs. = $0.88X$, or $X$ = 145.5 lbs. ÷ 0.88. Using a calculator to divide 145.5 by 0.88, you get an estimated optimal body weight of 165.3 pounds.

| WOMEN | | | | | | |
|---|---|---|---|---|---|---|
| GOAL | PERCENTILE | 20–29 | 30–39 | 40–49 | 50–59 | 60+ |
| | 99 | 5.4 | 7.3 | 11.6 | 11.6 | 15.4 |
| | 95 | 10.8 | 13.4 | 16.1 | 18.8 | 16.8 |
| | 90 | 14.5 | 15.5 | 18.5 | 21.6 | 21.1 |
| | 85 | 16.0 | 16.9 | 20.3 | 23.6 | 23.5 |
| IMPROVE **10%** | 80 | 17.1 | 18.0 | 21.3 | 25.0 | 25.1 |
| | 75 | 18.2 | 19.1 | 22.4 | 25.8 | 25.7 |
| | 70 | 19.0 | 20.0 | 23.5 | 26.6 | 27.5 |
| | 65 | 19.8 | 20.8 | 24.3 | 27.4 | 28.5 |
| IMPROVE TO **80%** | 60 | 20.6 | 21.6 | 24.9 | 28.5 | 29.3 |
| | 55 | 21.3 | 22.4 | 25.5 | 29.2 | 29.9 |
| | 50 | 22.1 | 23.1 | 26.4 | 30.1 | 30.9 |
| | 45 | 22.7 | 24.0 | 27.3 | 30.8 | 31.8 |
| | 40 | 23.7 | 24.9 | 28.1 | 31.6 | 32.5 |
| | 35 | 24.4 | 26.0 | 29.0 | 32.6 | 33.0 |
| | 30 | 25.4 | 27.0 | 30.1 | 33.5 | 34.3 |
| | 25 | 26.6 | 28.1 | 31.1 | 34.3 | 35.5 |
| IMPROVE **25%** | 20 | 27.7 | 29.3 | 32.1 | 35.6 | 36.6 |
| | 15 | 29.8 | 31.0 | 33.3 | 36.6 | 38.0 |
| | 10 | 32.1 | 32.8 | 35.0 | 37.9 | 39.3 |
| | 5 | 35.4 | 35.7 | 37.8 | 39.6 | 40.5 |
| | 1 | 40.5 | 40.0 | 45.5 | 50.8 | 47.0 |

## MORE GUIDELINES FOR FINDING
## YOUR OPTIMAL BODY-FAT PERCENTAGE

### 1ST–35TH PERCENTILES

**If your current body-fat percentage** places you between the 1st and 35th percentiles for your age and gender group, you might still be able to reach the 80th percentile eventually, but you might not, so it's best to set a more modest goal. Don't feel bad, though, because in another respect your goal can be more ambitious than those of athletes who are already relatively lean. Because your body carries a greater amount of excess fat, you can expect to sharply lower your body-fat percentage through proper training and diet. If you are currently between the 1st and 35th percentiles, your initial goal should be to move up five rows on Table 2.1. So if you're a 26-year-old female and your current body-fat percentage is 28.0, placing you in the 20th percentile for women aged 20 to 29, your initial goal is to move up five rows to the 45th percentile, at 22.7 percent body fat.

### 75TH–90TH PERCENTILES

**Those near the lean end** of the body composition continuum, meaning those whose current body-fat percentage places them at or above the 75th percentile for their reference group, cannot expect to lose much more body fat, but they can still expect to make big performance gains in losing a little body fat. If your current body-fat percentage is between the 75th and 90th percentiles, set an initial goal to move up just one or two rows on Table 2.1. Two rows represent an acceptable goal if you're currently rather far from peak race shape and/or your diet leaves much to be desired; one row is more realistic if you're already quite fit and eating healthily.

### 95TH–99TH PERCENTILES

**Athletes whose current body-fat percentage** places them in the 95th or 99th percentile for their age and gender should not set goals to lose any more of what little body fat they have, although they might become a bit leaner still in the process of becoming race fit. If you are already leaner than 95 out of 100 active persons your age, it is best to determine your optimal body composition using the functional method described in Chapter 7, where changes in body weight and body composition are plotted against changes in performance to identify racing weight prospectively.

## RACING WEIGHT CHEAT SHEET

**1** Step on a scale to get your current body weight and body-fat percentage.

**2** Determine your lean body mass by using these numbers and referring to Table 2.1. Calculate your current lean body-mass percentage by subtracting your current body-fat percentage from 100 percent (e.g., 100 – body-fat percentage).

*lean* BODY MASS =
CURRENT WEIGHT × *current lean* BODY-MASS PERCENTAGE

**3** To estimate your optimal bodyweight, use your lean body mass and estimated body-fat percentage. Calculate your optimal lean body-mass percentage by subtracting your optimal body-fat percentage from 100 percent (e.g., 100 – body-fat percentage).

OPTIMAL WEIGHT =
*lean* BODY MASS ÷ *optimal lean* BODY-MASS PERCENTAGE

This method of using an estimated optimal body-fat percentage to calculate an estimated optimal body weight will be less accurate for individuals who are likely to gain some lean body mass—namely, muscle—in the process of getting in shape. That's because gaining muscle lowers body-fat percentage even in the absence of body-fat loss. If you plan to do more weightlifting than you have in the recent past as part of your training, you can expect to gain a pound or two of muscle even as you lose fat and should account for this expected muscle weight gain in your estimated optimal body weight.

# TRUST THE PROCESS

Imagine starting a race without knowing where the finish line is. If you're like most endurance athletes, you won't like that. We are very finish-line focused. At the same time, most endurance athletes have a strong appreciation for process—all of the hard work that gets us to the starting line. I don't think there's a more patient breed of athlete. Runners, triathletes, and others of this ilk routinely put in months of training for a single opportunity to enjoy the thrill of crossing a finish line.

Your racing weight is, for better or worse, like a race with an unknown finish line. While you can estimate your racing weight before you ever reach it, to discover that weight, you must eat and train right for an extended period of time and see where these practices lead you. In other words, you must free yourself from your finish-line focus and concentrate on the process. It's time now to define this process, first of all by distinguishing performance weight management from dieting.

# THREE

# DIETING VS. PERFORMANCE WEIGHT MANAGEMENT

E veryone knows what a diet is. The concepts and methods of dieting are drilled into us from an early age. Most of us try dieting at some point in our lives, many of us more than once. Because dieting is so familiar and ubiquitous, we don't usually define it, but if we wanted to do so anyway, we could describe it as the practice of adopting a set of dietary rules—which usually include reduced food intake or forbidden food types—for the sake of losing weight.

For many, the road to becoming an endurance athlete began with a diet. Maybe this is your story. The guy who once had regularly ordered the bacon burger was suddenly rolling out special requests at a restaurant—keep the toast dry, hold the dressing, boil the egg, steam the vegetables. For most successful athletes, somewhere along the way a new lifestyle emerged and the focus shifted from dieting to performance.

Performance weight management is rather different from dieting. It is best defined as an ongoing effort to improve endurance performance by optimizing body composition for racing through nutritional, as well as other, means. Successful performance weight management usually results in the loss of body fat and body weight, but not always, because this is not, in fact, the goal. Some athletes attain their optimal racing weight by gaining muscle, for example.

Dieting can be an effective way to lose weight. Men and women who follow a traditional weight-loss diet such as Weight Watchers (based on calorie restriction) or the Atkins diet (based on food-type prohibition) often lose weight quickly at first. Unfortunately, however, few dieters stick with their program long enough to reach their weight goal, and more than 80 percent of those who do reach that goal through dieting eventually gain back most or all of the weight they lost.

Many endurance athletes use dieting to lose weight as well. But dieting is not really appropriate for endurance athletes. The goal of dieting—weight loss for its own sake—is not the proper goal for cyclists, runners, swimmers, and triathletes. Improved performance is the proper goal. While weight loss in endurance athletes is frequently associated with improved performance, it isn't always. When endurance athletes lose weight through dieting, their performance often suffers. The main problem is that the typical weight-loss diet fails to supply enough energy to support hard training. Diets based on food-type prohibitions sometimes also deprive the body of specific nutrients—especially carbohydrate—that are needed to properly absorb a heavy training load.

The most successful endurance athletes seldom diet, and except in special circumstances, they rarely try to lose weight. Instead, they manage their weight for performance through the various methods that make up the Racing Weight system: maximizing diet quality, managing appetite, balancing energy sources, monitoring performance, timing nutrient intake, and training smartly. The reason the most successful endurance athletes practice performance weight management instead of dieting is tautological. The common methods of performance weight management work—they improve performance—and are therefore more or less required for sustained success in endurance sports. Dieting, in contrast, tends to sabotage performance, making sustained competitive success difficult or impossible.

One of the greatest barriers to the attainment of an athlete's racing weight and the performance boost that comes with it is the dieting mind-set that our culture tries to instill in all of us. This mind-set is not necessarily an impediment to overweight nonathletes seeking quick weight loss, but it is an obstacle for endurance athletes who should be seeking improved performance through the optimization of their body composition for racing. If you're like most endurance athletes, you've been trained in the dieting mind-set more deeply than you realize. My goal

**TABLE 3.1 DIETING VERSUS PERFORMANCE WEIGHT MANAGEMENT**

| | DIETING | PERFORMANCE WEIGHT MANAGEMENT |
|---|---|---|
| **GOAL** | » Weight loss | » Improved performance through optimization of body composition |
| **METHODS** | » Reduced food intake<br>» Forbidden food prohibitions | » Increased diet quality<br>» Balanced energy sources<br>» Appetite management<br>» Self-monitoring<br>» Nutrient timing<br>» Smart training |
| **ATTEMPTED BY** | » Overweight persons<br>» Most age-group endurance athletes | » Successful endurance athletes |
| **APPROPRIATE FOR** | » Overweight persons | » All endurance athletes |
| **PROS** | » Rapid weight loss for some | » Long-term effectiveness<br>» Sustainability |
| **CONS** | » Hard to sustain<br>» Dismal long-term success rate<br>» Harmful to endurance performance | » Results too slow for some |

here is to undo that training and replace it with an appreciation for the performance weight management strategy that the most successful athletes depend on instead of dieting.

Table 3.1 provides a summary of the key differences between dieting and performance weight management.

# RUNNING ON EMPTY

Men and women who choose to diet for weight loss generally follow one of two paths. One path is a "diet with a name." There are hundreds of these, including the Zone Diet, Jenny Craig, and the China Diet. The other path is a diet a person devises for himself, such as eliminating soft drinks and not eating after 7:00 at night. Despite the apparent variety of the branded and do-it-yourself diets, all of them work (when they do work) the same way: by creating energy deficits. Consuming fewer calories than the body needs to maintain its current weight is the *only* way to lose weight. Eliminating food types, eating according to the glycemic index, maintaining specific macronutrient balances, and following other such rules are just so many ways of disguising a reduction in energy intake, without which weight loss can't happen.

A number of years ago scientists at the American Institute of Cancer Research (AICR) analyzed the nutritional guidelines presented in four diet books that were then popular: *Dr. Atkins' New Diet Revolution, The New Beverly Hills Diet, Protein Power,* and *Suzanne Somers' Get Skinny on Fabulous Food* (Meinz n.d.). None of these diets was promoted as a low-calorie diet. Each of them had its own distinct secret to weight loss. The secret of the New Beverly Hills Diet, for example, was food combining, whereas the secret of the Atkins diet was, of course, low carbohydrate intake. But the AICR analysis revealed that any reader who strictly followed the guidelines of any one of these four diets would in fact find herself on a low-calorie diet. Any weight loss that a person achieved on one of these programs would be attributable to the large calorie deficit it created, not to its proposed secret.

Other research has shown that the various popular weight-loss diets are more or less equally effective for overweight individuals who stick with them (Dansinger et al. 2005). This is only to be expected since, again, all such diets work the same way despite their disparate packaging. Endurance athletes are able to create even larger calorie deficits and lose weight even faster on traditional low-calorie diets because their training increases the amount of calories needed to maintain their current body weight. The catch—and it's a big one—is that large calorie deficits deprive the muscles of the fuel they need for optimal performance in workouts and for fast recovery between workouts.

The incompatibility of large energy deficits and intensive training was demonstrated in a 2009 study by a graduate student in exercise science at Southern Connecticut State University (Lunn, Finn, and Axtell 2009). A competitive cyclist himself, William Lunn compared the effects of sprint interval training, weight loss, and a combination of sprint interval training and weight loss on the power-weight ratio of experienced cyclists. The power-weight ratio is a measure of how much sustained power (measured in watts) an athlete can produce on a bike per kilogram or pound of body weight. It's considered one of the most important performance variables in cycling because it is a strong predictor of real-world competitive performance. The more watts per unit of weight an athlete can sustain, the faster he or she will go in races.

There are two ways to improve your power-to-weight ratio. One way is to increase sustained power output with improved fitness. The other is to lose weight.

Thirty-four cyclists participated in Lunn, Finn, and Axtell's study, and they were separated into four groups. For 10 weeks, one group's members added twice-weekly sprint interval sessions to their training to increase their power output while maintaining their current body weight, a second group continued with normal training while actively pursuing weight loss through dieting, a third group added sprint intervals and pursued weight loss, and a fourth, "control," group continued with normal training and maintained current body weight.

The results were revealing. Members of the sprint interval training group improved their power-weight ratio by an average of 10 percent. They achieved this gain entirely through an increase in their power output, as their weight did not change. Members of the weight-loss group increased their power-weight ratio almost as much—by an average of 9.3 percent. This gain was achieved entirely through weight loss (participants lost 11 lbs. on average), as their power output did not change. As you might expect, members of the control group experienced no gain in power, no weight loss, and thus no change in power-weight ratio.

But what might surprise you is that members of the combined sprint interval training and weight-loss group also did not improve their power-weight ratio over the 10-week study period. The problem for these individuals was that, while they did lose a significant amount of weight through dietary restriction, this very restriction seemed to prevent them from gaining any power through sprint interval training. More specifically, Lunn suggested, inadequate protein intake kept their muscles from adapting to the stress imposed by the sprints.

The general conclusion that Lunn and his colleagues drew from the results of the investigation was that cyclists seeking to enhance their power-weight ratio should *either* add sprint intervals to their training or lose weight, but should not do both simultaneously. This conclusion is consistent with the observation of many other exercise scientists, coaches, and athletes that the aggressive pursuit of weight loss through dietary restriction is not compatible with aggressive training for maximum performance. Maximum weight loss and maximum performance cannot be equal priorities for an endurance athlete at any given time.

There is, however, an appropriate time for endurance athletes to make weight loss a higher priority than performance, and that's when they are not actively training toward any upcoming races. One such time is the four- to eight-week period that follows an off-season break from training and precedes a formal return to race-focused training. Within this window it is appropriate to get a "quick start" back toward optimal racing weight with a relatively large energy deficit. Beginners may also choose to prioritize weight loss over performance before they do their first race. In Chapter 10 I will give you detailed guidelines on executing a quick start toward your racing weight either as a beginner or during the window between training cycles.

## SHRINKING THE ENGINE

Within the training cycle, it is important to avoid large energy deficits that harm performance. There are actually two distinct mechanisms by which this harm is done. Large energy deficits do not only rob the muscles of the fuel they need for optimal training performance. They also cause the athlete to lose muscle mass. Studies have shown that the larger the daily energy deficit is, the higher the ratio of muscle loss to fat loss becomes. One study found that with a daily energy deficit of 500 calories, only half of the weight that subjects lost was fat; the other half was lean body mass (Ball, Kyle, and Canary 1967). These results aren't desirable for anyone, but they are especially harmful to athletes whose muscles are their engines.

> MUSCLE TISSUE IS MORE THAN JUST THE BODY'S ENGINE; IT IS ALSO THE BODY'S FURNACE.

The consequences don't end there. Muscle tissue is more than just the body's engine; it is also the body's furnace. Even at rest the muscles gobble up energy. The amount of muscle mass on a person's body is the main determinant of his or her basal metabolic rate, or the number of calories that are burned throughout the day outside of workouts. Ironically, as muscle tissue is lost as a result of undereating for the sake of weight loss, it becomes harder to lose weight because the body is burning fewer and fewer calories.

## AN ELITE CASE STUDY

Many athletes have learned the hard way that aiming for large energy deficits is not the best way to shed excess body fat. One such athlete is Kara Goucher. Not long after she graduated from the University of Colorado as the winner of multiple NCAA titles in track and cross-country, Goucher suffered a knee injury that required surgery and left her completely unable to train for many weeks. Prone to weight gain during periods of downtime, Goucher put on 30 pounds of fat before her doctor finally released her to resume training.

Through a combination of training and improved diet, Goucher lost the first 20 pounds easily, but the last 10 were stubborn. Unable to shed them on her own, she sought help from sports nutritionist Dan Bernadot. An analysis of Goucher's diet revealed to Bernadot that she was eating roughly 1,200 calories a day. Calculations based on her height, weight, and training revealed that she needed approximately 2,400 calories a day. Bernadot explained to Goucher that her extreme energy deficit was causing her metabolism to slow to a crawl—the body's normal reaction to starvation—and that she actually needed to eat more to lose the rest of the fat she had accumulated during her convalescence.

Goucher had a hard time believing this explanation, but she lacked any better answers of her own, so she took a leap of faith and started eating more. The weight came off, and Goucher has avoided undereating ever since.

## A CASE STUDY CLOSER TO HOME

One of the reasons so few elite endurance athletes like Kara Goucher follow diets with names is that they have access to sports nutritionists like Dan Bernadot who steer them away from such diets. Age groupers tend to rely more on popular resources for guidance in weight management and are therefore more likely to find themselves stuck on low-calorie diets that sabotage their performance.

Many age-group endurance athletes, especially beginners, have a lot more weight to lose than any professional racer ever does. Since traditional dieting can result in rapid weight loss, age groupers who choose to follow a popular diet are often fooled initially into believing they are on the right path. Only when their weight loss tapers off and they discover that they feel terrible and perform poorly in all of their workouts do they realize something is wrong.

Kim Mueller, a San Diego–based sports nutritionist, has a lot of clients who come to her after running into a wall on some form of weight-loss diet. One such client, Juan Guevara, lost 60 pounds on a low-carb diet. A runner, Juan put his training on the back burner while he was focused on losing weight. But when he reached his weight-loss goal, Juan started to ramp up his workouts again in preparation for a half-marathon. Fearing that he might otherwise regain the weight he'd lost, Juan remained on his low-carb diet. The results were disastrous. When he came to Mueller's office, Juan reported that he felt sluggish in his runs and seemed to be getting nothing out of his training—his fitness was going nowhere. It was taking him forever to recover from harder runs, and he suffered from constant muscles aches and pains.

Mueller analyzed Juan's diet and learned that he was consuming only two-thirds as many calories as his body was using daily and was getting only half of the carbohydrate he needed. She corrected these imbalances, and a few months later she received the following e-mail from him: "I'm able to increase my run mileage and intensity without feeling like a bus ran me over and I just ran my fastest 13.1 in 10 years thanks to these dietary changes. I can't get over how quickly I'm recovering and how good I feel during workouts. And I haven't gained a pound!"

# THE SUSTAINABILITY FACTOR

If all's well that ends well, then perhaps Juan Guevara made no mistake in first losing weight with a low-calorie, low-carb diet and then improving his running by switching to a performance diet. After all, as I said above, there is a proper time for endurance athletes to prioritize weight-loss ahead of performance. However, even when weight loss is the top priority, it is better to pursue this objective through the rules of a Racing Weight quick start—which emulates how the most successful endurance athletes pursue rapid weight loss—than to follow a traditional weight-loss diet. That's because Juan Guevara is an exception. As I suggested earlier, in the majority of cases dieting not only sabotages performance but also fails to yield permanent weight loss.

The problem is that large calorie deficits produce persistent hunger, which is difficult to put up with for very long. Large calorie deficits are even harder on athletes than they are on nonathletes because of the effect of exercise on appetite. As the volume or intensity of exercise increases, appetite and food intake tend to increase as well. Research has shown that chronic exercise increases the sensitivity of the body's hormonal appetite-signaling system, stimulates unconscious changes in food preferences, and alters the pleasure response to food in ways that significantly boost daily calorie intake (Stensel 2010). Studies in which overweight, sedentary men and women have been placed on exercise programs have found that for every 10 calories a person burns through exercise, 3 more food calories are consumed as a result of increased appetite.

Scientists refer to the increase in food intake that follows upticks in exercise as the "compensation effect." The strength of this effect varies between individuals. Some people do not eat more even when their exercise level increases drastically, while others have been known to *gain* weight while training for marathons and triathlons. The leanest and swiftest endurance athletes are not necessarily immune to the compensation effect, however, nor do they actively resist it. As the elite athlete food journals presented in Chapter 12 will demonstrate, these people eat heartily. Yet they do not overeat. Instead of resisting their appetite, they manage it. Appetite management encompasses a variety of methods that are practiced widely by the most successful athletes and range from eating low-energy-density foods to avoiding "mindless eating," as we'll discuss in Chapter 5.

Hunger aside, most dieters start a diet with no intention of following its strict rules for life. The dieting mind-set is a short-term one. These days most popular diets present themselves as lifelong solutions, but few dieters approach them as such, and the severity of the privations they enforce makes it hard to bear the thought of adhering to them indefinitely. The plan for most dieters is to obey the rules until they reach their weight goal and then either go back to their old way of eating or loosen the restrictions they impose on themselves. As a result, many dieters succeed in reaching their weight goal and then gain back all of the weight they lost.

In contrast to dieting, performance weight management is truly a lifelong solution. Superficially, a quick start may look like a short-term diet that sets a person up to regain lost weight afterward. But the core "rules" of a quick start—including high diet quality and smart training—are the same as those governing race preparation.

Plus, insofar as the Racing Weight system does differ from the quick start, the latter does not leave the athlete high and dry. Most dieters have no plan for maintaining their weight loss after they achieve their weight goal and end their diet. Athletes who transition from a preseason or initial quick start to the Racing Weight system have a comprehensive plan in place. And that plan is both psychologically and physically more sustainable than a diet.

# ATHLETIC DIETING

There are some diets with names that are either tailored specifically to athletes or have caught on among athletes. The Zone Diet, which advocates a macronutrient breakdown of 40 percent carbs, 30 percent fat, and 30 percent protein, became popular among athletes in the late 1990s and is still used by some athletes today. The Paleo Diet, which requires its followers to eat as our Paleolithic ancestors presumably did a million years ago, is currently fashionable among endurance athletes and in the CrossFit crowd.

Such diets typically do not deprive athletes of the total calories they need to support their training. But like the popular weight-loss diets, they do tend to deprive athletes of adequate carbohydrate. Also, their restrictive, imbalanced nature makes them just as hard to sustain as low-calorie diets.

Research dating back almost a century has demonstrated that low-carb diets such as the Zone Diet reduce the body's capacity to handle higher training loads. In 2002, researchers at Kingston University in England looked at the effect of the Zone Diet on training capacity in runners (Jarvis et al. 2002). Volunteers were required to run as long as they could at a fixed intensity of 80 percent of $VO_2$ max on two separate occasions: before starting the Zone Diet and again after a week on the Zone Diet. The average time to exhaustion before the Zone Diet was 37:41. A week later the average time to exhaustion had dropped all the way down to 34:06. Just seven days of inadequate carb intake had reduced these runners' intensive endurance by nearly 10 percent.

Athletes who follow the Paleo Diet generally consume carbohydrates in amounts similar to Zone dieters because the Paleo Diet forbids the consumption of grains, which are nature's most concentrated source of carbs. We can expect therefore that the Paleo Diet has a similar effect on training capacity. But a greater problem with the Paleo Diet is its sheer restrictiveness. Not only are grains forbidden on this diet, but dairy products and legumes are as well. I, for one, could not remain a happy person for very long without bread and cheese in my life, and many athletes who try the Paleo Diet quickly discover that they cannot either.

## IT IS EASIER TO SUPPORT OPTIMAL PERFORMANCE WITH A MORE INCLUSIVE DIET.

If it were truly necessary to completely eliminate grains, dairy, and legumes from the diet to attain optimal racing weight, that would be one thing. But there is no evidence that this is the case. What's more, hard evidence in support of Paleo Diet creator Loren Cordain's belief that these foods types are bad for general health is also lacking. In fact, the best available evidence proves the opposite. We will discuss some of the benefits of the Paleo Diet's forbidden foods in the next chapter.

Any diet that forbids food types other than obvious junk foods such as candy is likely to be less nutritionally balanced, less healthful, and less supportive of endurance training than a more inclusive diet. Whole grains, legumes, and dairy foods have unique nutrient profiles that are not found in other types of foods. Some experts believe that the most disruptive imbalance in the Paleo Diet is not inadequate carbohydrate supply but rather excessive fiber intake, which impedes the absorption of vitamins and minerals.

Similarly, lean meats, fish, eggs, and dairy foods, which are eliminated from strict vegetarian diets, contain a number of nutrients—including amino acids and iron—that are helpful to endurance and less available in plant foods. This is not to say that a vegetarian diet cannot support optimal endurance performance, but it is easier to support optimal performance with a more inclusive diet. For example, iron deficiency is very common in high-level runners, especially in those runners who eat the least meat. There are many successful vegetarian endurance athletes. I would never tell an athlete who chooses to be vegetarian for ethical, visceral, or even aesthetic reasons not to do so. But I do not recommend that endurance athletes go vegetarian for the sake of weight management and performance alone.

## DOING WHAT WORKS

Another characteristic that all weight-loss diets share is the manner in which they are created. Each such diet's secret to weight loss is made up in someone's head and then tried out on the world to see if it works. As we've seen, most traditional weight-loss diets work reasonably well in the short term and not at all in the long term. Performance weight management was created in the opposite way. Through long-term, collective trial and error, successful endurance athletes have discovered a handful of methods for weight management and performance enhancement that always work. Far from inventing these methods, I've used my head simply to identify them so that I can pass them along to you.

Some interesting research has investigated the methods that actually work to produce permanent weight loss among men and women in the real world. Interestingly, most of these methods have nothing to do with what people eat per se. And some of these methods, including frequent self-monitoring, are also among the methods that endurance athletes use for successful performance weight management (Butryn et al. 2007).

Researchers have even gotten to the point where they can predict with a fair degree of accuracy who will defy the odds and achieve permanent weight loss through dieting. It's pretty simple, really. Those who believe most strongly that their diet will work and will be worth the sacrifices involved usually get the best long-term results. This attitude is also important for your effort to reach your optimal racing weight through the better approach of performance weight management. That's why I've taken the time in this chapter to spell out the crucial differences between dieting and performance weight management and explain why the latter is better. Now that you really believe in the Racing Weight program, it's time to learn the specifics of how to practice it.

# 6 STEPS
# TO PEAK
# PERFORMANCE

# PART II

# FOUR

STEP 1

# IMPROVING YOUR DIET QUALITY

T hrough the first decade and more of his long career as a professional cyclist, Chris Horner lived on a diet of Coca-Cola, Snickers bars, breakfast burritos, donuts, Little Debbie brownies and Swiss Rolls, hold-the-veggies sandwiches, potato chips, and fast food. Despite eating this way, Horner stayed lean and light at 150 pounds and excelled as a climbing specialist, winning numerous U.S. races. He saw no reason to fix what did not seem broken—until a crash in the 2009 Tour of California left him unable to ride for two weeks.

Fearing the rapid weight gain that would surely be his lot if he kept living on candy bars and soft drinks, Horner decided to finally give better eating a try. He drastically reduced his consumption of fast food and sweets and introduced fruits and vegetables to his diet. Even after he made these changes, his diet remained far from perfect, but it was much improved—and it made a difference.

Because Horner had always maintained a low body weight and a low body-fat percentage, he had always assumed he was already at his ideal racing weight. But after changing his diet, he learned otherwise. He dropped down to 140 pounds and as a result began climbing better than ever. The 2010 season, when he was 38 years old, was one of the best of his career, highlighted by his first victory in a European stage race—the Tour of the Basque Country.

What's interesting about the diet changes that led to Horner's weight loss and improved performance is their simplicity. Any fifth-grader knows that candy bars and soft drinks are fattening and that fruits and vegetables are slimming. Common sense told Horner that if he had less of the fattening foods in his diet and added some slimming foods, he would lose weight—or at least avoid gaining weight during the two weeks when he was unable to ride his bike. There was no need to count calories or learn the glycemic index of whatever he considered putting in his mouth or complicating the process in any other way. All Horner really did was improve the overall quality of his diet.

## WEIGHT MANAGEMENT MADE SIMPLE

A year after Horner won his first European stage race, a study from the Harvard School of Public Health validated his commonsense approach to dietary weight management (Mozaffarian et al. 2011). It proved that eating fewer fattening foods and more slimming foods is critical to weight management not just for professional cyclists but also for everyone.

The study included data on eating habits and changes in body weight collected from more than 120,000 men and women over a period of 20 years. The researchers looked at how consumption of just a few, specific high-quality and low-quality foods affected patterns of weight change over time. The average subject gained 16.8 pounds over 20 years. Data analysis revealed that almost all of this weight gain was associated with frequent consumption of low-quality foods such as potato chips and was negated by frequent consumption of high-quality foods such as vegetables.

For example, each daily serving of potato chips was linked to 1.69 lbs. of weight gain every four years. By contrast, each daily serving of nuts was associated with a 0.57-lb. attenuation of weight gain over four years.

It might be tempting to dismiss this study as a case of proving the obvious. Of course people who eat a lot of potato chips gain more weight over time! But the keys to effective weight management—for nonathletes and athletes alike—have always been obvious. The reason so many of us struggle with weight management is that we don't do the obvious.

| THE AVERAGE PERSON GAINED | THE COST OF LOW-QUALITY FOODS: | THE REWARD OF HIGH-QUALITY FOODS: |
|---|---|---|
| **0.84** LBS. *annually in* **20** years. | 1 daily serving of potato chips = **1.69** LBS. *of extra weight every* **4** years. | 1 daily serving of nuts = **-0.57** LBS. *of weight loss every* **4** years. |

Instead, we reach beyond the obvious for magic bullets and revolutionary new miracle solutions that promise to make weight management easy but never deliver on that promise.

What the Harvard study reveals is that, although effective weight management may never be easy, it can at least be simple—simpler than tallying fat grams or looking up the gluten content of everything you consider eating. Again, the average fifth-grader knows the difference between high-quality and low-quality foods. With this knowledge and a little discipline, you can identify a few high-quality foods to eat more of and a few low-quality foods to eat less of and thereby attain and sustain your optimal racing weight.

Improving your diet quality is the first step of the Racing Weight plan because it is the single most effective way to get leaner—and the simplest. If you did only one thing to shed excess body fat, adding high-quality foods to and subtracting low-quality foods from your diet would be the way to go. Once you've elevated your diet quality, you will be well on your way toward attaining your racing weight. The other five steps of the Racing Weight plan will take you the rest of they way.

## MEASURING DIET QUALITY

When you think about the concept of quantifying how "good" or "bad" a person's diet is, the first thing that comes to mind is probably a tool such as the glycemic index (GI). But these familiar tools don't really measure the overall quality of a person's diet; instead they isolate one specific effect of food on the body among dozens of effects.

Twenty years ago most people had never heard of the glycemic index, which is a measure of how quickly the blood glucose level rises after carbohydrate-containing foods are consumed. Researchers began to focus on the glycemic index in the early 1980s. They found that the body processes equal amounts of high-GI and low-GI carbs quite differently and that these differences might have important implications for health. Their excitement gradually made its way out of the laboratory and into society at large.

In 2002, with the publication of *The New Glucose Revolution*, the glycemic index burst into the collective consciousness as the low-carb diet craze (which did not distinguish between high-GI and low-GI carbs) sank toward its inevitable demise. In the United States a new diet trend trumpeted the glycemic index as the new skeleton key of weight management. *The New Glucose Revolution* and the many similar books that followed it taught us that high-glycemic foods increase appetite, cause carbohydrate cravings and sugar addiction, promote fat storage, and lead to the development of diabetes.

There was never much proof that any of this was true, but subsequent research has made it quite clear that the glycemic index is a nearly useless tool for weight management or general health promotion. The essential problem with the glycemic index is that it isolates one characteristic of food, pulls it out of context, and blows it completely out of proportion. Notwithstanding the fact that key tenets of the GI philosophy (such as the notion that high-GI foods promote cravings for more high-GI foods) have been exposed as myths, the key weakness of the GI philosophy is that there's a lot more to food than its effect on blood glucose.

To draw an exercise analogy, using the glycemic index to guide your diet is a bit like using blood lactate measurements to control the intensity of your workouts. While there is a correlation between blood lactate levels and fatigue, recent studies have determined that there is no causal connection. Blood lactate levels just happen to increase in parallel to other muscle chemistry events that do cause fatigue. And since blood lactate is not only unconnected to fatigue but also tedious to measure, there's really no point in doing so.

Similarly, many of the low-quality, processed foods we eat today have high-GI values, while most of the high-quality natural foods we are meant to eat have low-GI values. Consequently, the average GI value of an individual's diet is, in fact, a somewhat reliable indicator of a diet's healthfulness. However, foods are not high or low quality *because of* their glycemic index. There is merely an association between properties that make certain foods high or low quality, such as fiber content, and their effect on blood glucose levels.

While the glycemic index is the metric that has distracted the most people from diet quality, there are many other examples, including the inflammatory index, which makes too much of the effects of various foods on systemic inflammation, and pH value (a measure of the acidity or alkalinity of a substance), which makes too much of the effects of various foods on body acidity. All such metrics suffer from the fact that they are too narrow. The only truly useful measure of a food's value is its total concentration and balance of nutrients. So how do we measure food and diet quality?

Before the last years of the twentieth century, research scientists focused primarily on the health effects of individual nutrients. The value of such studies was limited, however, because the health effects of individual nutrients depend heavily on the total dietary context in which they are consumed. Thus, a need arose to quantify the overall quality of a diet to reflect how people really eat.

Various diet-quality indices, including the Healthy Eating Index and the Diet Quality Index, have since been created. The Diet Quality Index has been described (Newby et al. 2003) as "a dietary assessment instrument based on 10 dietary recommendations reflecting dietary guidelines and policy in the United States." The original Diet Quality Index assigned scores in a range of 0 to 16 (where the lowest score was the best) based on the amount of eight different food and nutrient types present in the diet. These nutrients are total fat, saturated fat, cholesterol, fruit and vegetables, grains and legumes, protein, sodium, and calcium. Testing of the original index revealed that its effectiveness as a predictor of disease risk was limited by the fact that it did not consider these aspects of diet:

- **VARIETY:** A more varied diet tends to reduce disease risk,
- **PROPORTIONALITY:** The proportions of various nutrients and foods relative to one another matter.
- **MODERATION:** A diet that provides more calories than needed tends to increase disease risk regardless of where the calories come from.

Hence a revised index that incorporated these factors was created and has been used ever since.

While the Diet Quality Index is a useful tool in nutritional epidemiological studies, it is far too complex for the average layperson to use to monitor and control the quality of his or her own diet. During the past 15 years, nutrition scientists who recognized the potential value of a dietary-quality measurement tool for individual consumers, and the inadequacy of existing scientific tools for this purpose, have proposed various new metrics that do not require a doctorate to implement.

# THE DIET QUALITY SCORE

Not satisfied with any of the existing tools that individuals might use to manage their own dietary quality, I created the Diet Quality Score (DQS) several years ago (see Table 4.1 for how to score each food group and food serving). It works by assigning a score to your total eating for one day that is the sum of point values assigned to the individual items you eat throughout the day. The higher your DQS score, the healthier your diet is. The DQS represents a simple, practical, realistic, and holistic approach to measuring diet quality. It is a tool you can use as often as every day to generate an accurate picture of how healthily you're eating without making a significant commitment of time and energy.

The Diet Quality Score considers the intrinsic wholesomeness of foods as well as the factors of balance and moderation that also contribute to overall diet quality. Foods are divided into the following 10 categories: fruits, vegetables, lean meats and fish, nuts and seeds, whole grains, dairy, refined grains, sweets, fried foods, and fatty proteins. Foods in the first six of these categories are high quality and therefore add points to your daily DQS. Foods in the last four categories are low quality and therefore subtract points from your daily DQS. To determine your DQS for any given day, all you have to do is identify the category for each item you've eaten, find the point total assigned to that category, and tally the points.

The DQS encourages balanced eating through its use of six separate high-quality food categories. To maximize your daily DQS, you need to eat foods in all six of these categories, in part because the point value assigned to foods within any given category declines as you consume

**TABLE 4.1 HOW TO SCORE YOUR DIET QUALITY**

| | FOOD TYPE | SERVING NUMBER | | | | | |
|---|---|---|---|---|---|---|---|
| | | 1ST | 2ND | 3RD | 4TH | 5TH | 6TH |
| HIGH QUALITY | Fruits | 2 | 2 | 2 | 1 | 0 | 0 |
| | Vegetables | 2 | 2 | 2 | 1 | 0 | 0 |
| | Lean meats & fish | 2 | 2 | 1 | 0 | 0 | -1 |
| | Nuts & seeds | 2 | 2 | 1 | 0 | 0 | -1 |
| | Whole grains | 2 | 2 | 1 | 0 | 0 | -1 |
| | Dairy | 1 | 1 | 1 | 0 | -1 | -2 |
| LOW QUALITY | Refined grains | -1 | -1 | -2 | -2 | -2 | -2 |
| | Sweets | -2 | -2 | -2 | -2 | -2 | -2 |
| | Fried foods | -2 | -2 | -2 | -2 | -2 | -2 |
| | Fatty proteins | -1 | -1 | -2 | -2 | -2 | -2 |

*Note:* See Table 13.1, page 236, for a version of this table that has been adapted for vegetarian/vegan diets.

more servings of them throughout any single day. For example, your first, second, and third daily servings of dairy add 1 point each to your score, but your fourth serving adds none, your fifth serving subtracts 1, and your sixth serving subtracts 2. This feature of the DQS reflects the fact that it is possible to consume too much of any food no matter how nutritious. The declining point value of high-quality foods with multiple servings also encourages *moderation*, because it ensures that you cannot indefinitely increase your DQS simply by eating more.

The DQS approach to diet-quality assessment has been indirectly validated by a large study conducted by Swedish researchers (Michels and Wolk 2002). The authors of this study divided foods into "healthy" and "unhealthy" categories very much like the high-quality and low-quality categories of the DQS. The diets of more than 58,000 women were analyzed for the variety of healthy and unhealthy foods they contained. The researchers discovered that those women who ate the greatest *variety* of healthy foods had the lowest mortality rate over a 10-year period, while those who ate the greatest variety of unhealthy foods had the highest mortality rate.

# DQS FOOD CATEGORIES

Before I give you specific guidelines on using the Diet Quality Score, let me first define and explain the 10 food categories. I will be the first to admit that strictly defining some food categories as high quality and others as low quality is somewhat artificial. In truth, I don't think it's quite accurate to classify any food category as low quality. A can of soda could save your life in the right circumstances, for example. Going even further, I don't like the nearly universal practice of distinguishing some nutrients as "good" and others as "bad." By definition, a nutrient is a chemical compound that the body can use to keep itself functioning. Therefore, all nutrients are good in one sense. Consider the example of saturated fat. This nutrient is widely considered to be bad, but the human body uses saturated fats in all kinds of helpful ways. Saturated fat is good. It just so happens that the modern diet contains too much of it. In most cases, what we really mean when we label a certain nutrient bad is that we tend to consume it in excess.

## IMPROVING THE QUALITY OF YOUR DIET

The logic by which I developed the high-quality and low-quality food categories of the DQS was this: I wanted a set of categories that would, in a practical, if not a scientifically rigorous, way, encourage individuals to consume enough of the nutrients (such as fiber) that most of us do not consume enough of and to consume fewer of the nutrients (such as sugar) that we typically consume in excess. I don't really believe that meats that are slightly more than 10 percent fat are low quality and that meats that are slightly less than 10 percent fat are high quality in any rigorous sense. I do, however, believe that designating them as such is a helpful way to promote more balanced nutrition.

With respect to weight management, quality is a function of three specific attributes of a food type: naturalness, calorie density, and nutrient density. Of these, naturalness is the most important.

Naturalness has to do mainly with how long a type of food has been a part of the human diet. The longer our species has been eating a type of food, the more natural it is for us and the more favorably it affects our body (including our body composition). Naturalness also refers to the relative "wholeness" of a specific food. Foods are more whole when they are less processed or modified from their natural state. For example, refined wheat flour is less "whole" than whole-wheat flour and therefore less natural. Likewise, processed meats such as many cold cuts are less whole than unprocessed meats, especially those from grass-fed livestock.

As we've seen, foods that are less calorie dense are less likely to promote weight gain. Natural foods tend to be less calorie dense than processed foods, but there are exceptions. Yet natural foods are less likely to promote weight gain even when they are more calorie dense than processed foods. For example, nuts are more calorie dense than white bread, yet they are "slimming," whereas white bread is fattening.

Research has shown that when people add more nutrient-dense foods (or foods with higher concentrations of vitamins, minerals, and phytonutrients) to their diets, they become less hungry, eat less, and lose weight (or gain it more slowly) (Fuhrman et al. 2010). This doesn't mean you can throw a bunch of powdered vitamins, minerals, and antioxidants into a blender with water, drink it, and expect to stay full until your next mealtime. Natural foods tend to be more nutrient dense than processed foods, but even when they're not, they have a stronger effect on hunger, eating, and body weight.

Neither energy density nor nutrient density can be considered independently of naturalness in assessing the quality of a food type.

## COUNTING YOUR SERVINGS

To use the DQS effectively, you need to know how to count servings for the various food types listed in the DQS table. With high-quality foods, I believe in using commonsense guidelines for serving sizes that are based on the amounts we typically eat. While it is often said that we tend to eat excessively large portions these days, this is typically not the case with high-quality foods such as vegetables and whole grains. The thing to watch out for is counting too small a portion of a high-quality food as a serving. A packet of ketchup does not count as a vegetable serving (and not because it's technically a fruit)! In the following sections I present commonsense serving-size guidelines for each of the 10 food categories. While I do define serving sizes for low-quality foods, any amount of an unhealthy food (within reason—you don't have to count a single sip of soda or two french fries) counts as a serving. I define serving sizes for low-quality foods in this way so that you will be sure to count your portions of such foods as two servings when you consume more than one serving's worth of them!

## HIGH-QUALITY FOODS

Here's the basic information you need to know about the six high-quality food categories.

### Fruits

The fruit category includes whole fresh fruits, canned and frozen fruits, and 100 percent fruit juices. Commonsense fruit serving sizes include one medium-size piece of whole fruit (e.g., one whole banana), a big handful of berries, and a medium-size glass of 100 percent fruit juice. Fruits are considered high quality because they are rich in a variety of essential vitamins and minerals. In addition, fruits are packed with 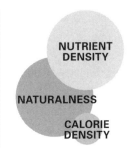 technically nonessential nutrients, known as phytonutrients, that function as antioxidants in the body. Until recently it was believed that phytonutrients functioned in the same way as the body's endogenous antioxidants, such as glutathione, which directly neutralize free radicals. Now it is believed that phytonutrients are actually weak toxins that stimulate the body's endogenous antioxidants through a stress reaction, much as other positive stressors such as exercise strengthen various systems of the body. In any case, we know that men and women who consume high levels of fruits exhibit higher antioxidant capacities, are less prone to chronic diseases, and live longer.

Fruits also contain a lot of fiber and water and relatively few calories. The effect of a food on hunger is determined primarily by its volume and only secondarily by the calories within it. Fiber and water add volume to foods without adding calories. Consequently, they have a high satiety index, which means that they provide a relatively large degree of hunger satisfaction per calorie and promote a lean body composition. The health benefits of fruit consumption are optimized at an intake level of three to four servings per day, as reflected in the Diet Quality Score.

Note that fruit juice counts as fruit in government and other official dietary guidelines. This is a controversial assessment, however, because fruit juices do not contain all of the nutrients in the whole fruits they come from. For example, most of the flavonoids (antioxidants) in oranges are contained in the pulp, very little of which makes its way into orange juice. Thus, while 100 percent fruit juices are more nutritious than most beverages, I do not recommend that you rely on them to meet your daily fruit requirements.

## Vegetables

The vegetable category of the DQS includes whole, fresh vegetables eaten cooked or raw, canned and frozen vegetables, and pureed or liquefied vegetables used in soups, sauces, and such. Commonsense vegetable serving sizes are a fist-sized portion of solid veggies, a half cup of tomato sauce, and a medium-sized bowl of vegetable soup or salad.

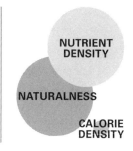

Like fruits, vegetables are loaded with vitamins, minerals, and phytonutrients; contain large amounts of fiber and water; and are relatively low in calories, so they provide nearly everything your body needs to function healthily and promote a lean body composition. The benefits of eating vegetables, like those of fruit, are maximized at an intake level of three to four servings per day.

## Lean Meats & Fish

Included in the lean meats and fish category are all types of fish and meats that are 10 percent fat or less. A commonsense serving of meat or fish is the size of your open hand.

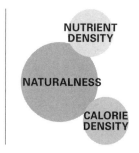

Epidemiological studies such as the one from the Harvard School of Public Health that I described earlier in the chapter have generally found that people who eat more meat tend to gain more weight in the long term, while people who eat more fish tend to gain less weight. I believe that if a study were to look at consumption of lean meats specifically, it would find that their effect on body weight is similar to that of fish.

Both fish and lean meats support a lean body composition because they are high in protein, which is the most satiating macronutrient calorie for calorie and is also less readily converted to body fat than fats and carbohydrates. Fish and lean meats are also good sources of a variety of vitamins and minerals, including vitamin B12 and iron.

Examples of lean meats and fish include beef tenderloin, water-packed canned tuna, skinless chicken breasts, wild-caught fish, extra-lean ground beef, extra-lean ground turkey, London broil, lean roast beef, turkey breast, leg of lamb, and pork tenderloins. Eggs can be counted as a lean meat despite their high fat content. People who eat eggs regularly tend to be slightly leaner than people who don't.

## Nuts & Seeds

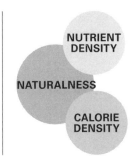

The original DQS system lumped nuts and seeds together with lean meats and fish in a category labeled "lean proteins." I've since given nuts and seeds their own category because their nutritional profile is really rather different from that of meat and fish and because it seemed counterintuitive for animal foods and plant foods to share a single category. The nuts and seeds category includes all the commonly eaten varieties of nuts and seeds as well as natural nut butters (without added sugar), such as peanut butter and almond butter.

Nuts and seeds contain a highly satiating combination of proteins and healthy unsaturated fats. It is not surprising, then, that research (Bes-Rastrollo et al. 2009) suggests people who eat a lot of nuts tend to have slightly lower than average body weights. A commonsense serving of nuts or seeds is a palmful. A commonsense serving of any nut butter is a heaping tablespoon.

## Whole Grains

The whole-grain category includes brown rice and breakfast cereals, breads, and pastas made with 100 percent whole grains. Commonsense servings of whole grains are a fist-sized portion of brown rice, a medium-sized bowl of cereal or pasta, and two slices of bread.

Even though some nutrition experts encourage minimal consumption of any and all grains, because they are less nutrient dense and more calorie dense than vegetables, I believe that whole grains have a place in the endurance athlete's diet because they are rich sources of carbohydrate, which is the energy source that endurance athletes need most. Whole grains have more fiber, vitamins, and minerals than refined grains, such as white rice. Whole grains also support a lean body composition. Studies have shown that individuals who consume the greatest amount of whole grains are less likely to be overweight than those who eat fewer whole grains (Good et al. 2008). This is in part because whole-grain calories are more filling, so those who tend to choose whole grains over refined grains eat less overall, and because the body uses more energy to digest whole grains than refined grains.

## Dairy

My original DQS system categorized low-fat dairy as a high-quality food group and whole-milk dairy as a low-quality food group. I've since tweaked the system so that all dairy foods are categorized as a high-quality food group. The reason is that there is no difference between the long-term effects of whole-milk dairy and low-fat dairy on body weight. All forms of dairy tend to limit long-term weight gain. In fact, the

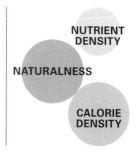

NUTRIENT DENSITY

NATURALNESS

CALORIE DENSITY

Harvard School of Public Health study found that yogurt attenuated long-term weight gain better than any other food, including fruits and vegetables.

Indeed, because whole-milk dairy is less processed than low-fat dairy, it is arguably a higher-quality food. It is not a food's effect on body composition alone that determines its quality. Its total nutrient content and its naturalness also count. Remember, all six categories of high-quality food are distinguished by their naturalness, high nutrient density, and beneficial effects on body composition.

Dairy foods support a lean body composition through their high protein content and also their high calcium content. Calcium reduces the activity of a hormone called calcitriol that promotes fat storage.

Dairy foods encompass all foods made with milk, including milk itself. Goat and sheep's milk count as well as cow's milk. Commonsense servings of dairy include a glass of milk or the amount of milk you'd normally use in a bowl of breakfast cereal, two slices of deli cheese, and a single-serving tub of yogurt.

Dairy foods that contain added sugar—including ice cream, frozen yogurt, some nonfrozen yogurts, and many flavored milk products—should be double-counted as dairy foods and sweets.

## LOW-QUALITY FOODS

Here's the basic information you need to know about the four low-quality food categories.

### Refined Grains

The category of refined grains includes white rice, processed flours, and all breakfast cereals, pastas, breads, and other baked goods made with less than 100 percent whole grains. Commonsense servings are the same as they are for the whole-grains category—a fist-sized portion of white rice, a medium-sized bowl of cereal or pasta, and two slices of bread.

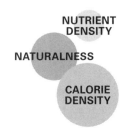

Refined grains are classified as low-quality foods in the Diet Quality Score because they contain more calories and provide less satiety than whole grains. There are 100 percent whole-grain varieties of every grain-based food you might care to eat, from bagels to ziti, so it just makes sense whenever possible to choose them instead of varieties made with refined grains.

### Sweets

This category includes all foods and beverages containing large amounts of refined sugars, including soft drinks, candy, pastries, and other desserts. If you're unsure about whether a certain food or beverage should be counted as a sweet, use the second-ingredient rule: If any type of refined sugar (which includes brown rice syrup, brown sugar, corn syrup, dextrose, fructose, high fructose corn syrup, maltose, sucrose, and sugar) is listed as the first or second ingredient, it's a sweet.

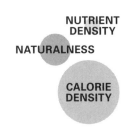

Even though they do not contain sugar, diet soft drinks sweetened artificially should also be counted as sweets. Studies have shown that regular consumption of diet sodas causes as much long-term weight gain as a daily habit of drinking regular soft drinks. The reason appears to be that artificial sweeteners alter brain chemistry to promote overeating.

Here's the good news: Dark chocolate does not count as a sweet if it's at least 80 percent cacao and eaten in small amounts (no more than 100 calories' worth at a time). One serving a day of dark chocolate need not be scored because it contains less sugar than most sweets and is rich in heart-healthy antioxidants.

Sweets other than dark chocolate are classified as low-quality foods because they are a major source of excess calories in the American diet. Seventeen percent of the average American's calories come from sugars. That's ridiculous. Sweets promote body-fat accumulation more than any

**17%**
of the **CALORIES**
consumed by the
average person
come from
*SUGARS*

## SWEETS IN DISGUISE

**I didn't have to wander far** in my local grocery store to find examples of everyday foods that must be counted as sweets in the DQS system because some form of sugar is their second (or even first) ingredient. Each of these foods is to be scored as another food type as well. For example, Mott's Apple Sauce is a fruit and a sweet.

| EVERYDAY FOODS | SUGAR INGREDIENT |
| --- | --- |
| Apple Sauce, Mott's | High Fructose Corn Syrup |
| Beef Jerky, Oh Boy! Oberto Teriyaki | Brown Sugar |
| Blueberry Muffins, Fiber One | Sugar (1st ingredient) |
| Cheerios, General Mills Honey Nut | Sugar |
| Dried Blueberries, Kirkland | Sugar |
| Granola Bars, Nature Valley Sweet & Salty Nut | High Maltose Corn Syrup |
| Oatmeal, Archer Farms Cherry Almond Instant (Organic) | Organic Dehydrated Cane Juice Solids |
| Tomato Soup, Campbell's | High Fructose Corn Syrup |
| Yogurt, Yoplait Strawberry | Sugar |

I'm not suggesting you need to swear off tomato soup and granola bars. But do read the list of ingredients a little more carefully. And remember, just because something is organic doesn't mean that it passes the second-ingredient test!

other type of food because they are extremely calorie dense and provide relatively little satiety.

Commonsense serving sizes of sweets include one small cookie, 12 ounces of soft drink, one label-defined serving of candy or (less than 80 percent cacao) chocolate, one regular-sized slice of pie or cake, and a scoop or bowl of ice cream.

## Fried Foods

This category includes all deep-fried foods such as potato chips, fried chicken, fried meats, and donuts. All snack chips except popped corn are in this category, including those that are not fried and even those made with vegetables other than potatoes and corn. The differences in calories are typically marginal, as are the differences in nutrient density. Snack chips just aren't a category of food you want to rely on when you're trying to get leaner.

NUTRIENT DENSITY

NATURALNESS

CALORIE DENSITY

The fried foods category does not include pan-fried foods such as stir-fries and fried eggs. Commonsense servings of fried foods include one small bag of potato chips, one fried hamburger patty, three or four buffalo wings, one small bag of chips, one small order of french fries, and one donut.

Deep frying adds a ton of calories to the base foods being fried. For example, a 156-gram baked potato contains roughly 145 calories, whereas a medium serving of french fries (117 grams) contains 387 calories. The oils used in frying are some of the most calorie dense foods in existence. Including fried foods in your diet is a surefire way to gain excess body fat. Eat as few of them as your cravings will allow!

| HIGH-QUALITY: | LOW-QUALITY: |
|---|---|
| **156 g** | **1** |
| baked potato = | medium serving of french fries = |
| **145** | **387** |
| *calories* | *calories* |

### Fatty Proteins

Fatty proteins are meats containing more than 10 percent fat as well as farm-raised fish. Fatty-protein serving sizes are the same as low-fat meat serving sizes—enough meat to fit in your open hand. Examples of fatty proteins include bacon, beef ribs, bologna and most other cold cuts, tuna packed in oil, chicken with skin, regular ground beef, regular ground turkey, farm-

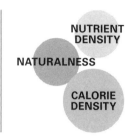

raised fish, ham, most cuts of lamb, prime cut beef, pork chops, pork ribs, rib eye steaks, salami, most sausages, T-bone steaks, and veal.

## SCORING COMMON FOODS

### Combination Foods

Many of the foods we commonly eat contain foods from multiple categories. How should these be scored? Use commonsense servings to score the constituent parts of the combination food individually. For example, suppose you have a few slices of pepperoni pizza. Count the crust as one serving of refined grain, the tomato sauce as half a vegetable serving, the cheese as one serving of dairy, and the pepperoni as one serving of fatty protein.

### Condiments, Sauces, and Spreads

Condiments, sauces, and spreads generally add a substantial number of calories to foods without contributing much to their satiating effect. Thus, they could be considered their own class of low-quality foods. When used sparingly on otherwise high-quality foods, they don't do any harm, so don't score them at all. But if you dip your french fries in mayonnaise or smoother your pork ribs in barbecue sauce, apply a –1 score to the mayonnaise or barbecue sauce in addition to subtracting 2 points from your DQS for the french fries or ribs.

Of course, some foods in this category are not low quality. If you snack on tortilla chips with homemade guacamole, for example, count the guacamole as a vegetable because it's typically made from nothing but vegetables (although avocado is technically a fruit) and spices.

Bear in mind that DQS is a created phenomenon, not a discovered phenomenon, so there is not a single right way to score every food. If you do the best you can to score complex foods such as stews and casseroles fairly, this tool will work as it's intended.

### Alcohol, Coffee, and Tea

In moderation, alcohol consumption has a positive effect on cardiovascular health and no long-term effect on body weight. Do not score your first alcoholic drink of the day if you're female or your first two if you're male. Each additional drink earns a –2 score, however, because drinking beyond moderation is much worse than not drinking at all.

Coffee and tea are also good for heart health owing to their antioxidant content. Do not score any coffee or tea you drink if you drink it unsweetened or lightly sweetened. If you drink lattes or other coffee- or tea-based drinks with a lot of milk, creamer, or sugary syrup, apply a score of –1 or –2 depending on the size and what you have added.

### Ergogenic Aids

What about sports drinks, carbohydrate gels, energy bars, and other ergogenic aids? Anything you consume during exercise should not be included in your daily DQS as the normal rules of food quality are suspended during exercise. Research has shown that when athletes take in calories during exercise, they consume fewer calories afterward, so the calories in ergogenic aids are truly negated.

Many endurance athletes frequently snack on energy bars outside of exercise. Those bars that are made primarily from whole grains and other natural foods such as nuts and fruit (Clif Bar) should be scored as follows: first serving: +1; second serving: –1; additional servings: –2. The reason is that even the healthiest energy bars provide a limited nutrient profile, are very calorie dense, and have a low satiety index, so they quickly turn from a positive to a negative when relied on too heavily during the day. Energy bars that are essentially candy bars in disguise (PowerBar Triple Threat) should be scored as follows: first serving: –1; any additional servings: –2.

# PUTTING DQS INTO PRACTICE

Now that you know how to calculate a one-day Diet Quality Score, it's time to use the DQS to improve your diet. The first step is to calculate an initial score to establish a baseline. Write down everything you eat over the course of one day, determine the food types and the number of servings represented, and add up your positive and negative points. Having established your baseline, find ways to increase your DQS.

There are three ways to do so: (1) eliminate low-quality foods from your diet, (2) add high-quality foods, and (3) replace low-quality foods with high-quality substitutes. I recommend that you start by making substitutions. Eliminating low-quality foods is not the best way to start in most cases because it tends to reduce dietary satisfaction. By replacing low-quality foods with high-quality alternatives, you maintain a steady level of eating while reducing excesses in sugar, fat, and total calories. It's the least disruptive way to improve your diet quality. Table 4.2 illustrates

**TABLE 4.2 HOW TO IMPROVE YOUR DAILY DQS**

| | TYPICAL | DQS | BETTER | DQS |
|---|---|---|---|---|
| **BREAKFAST** | » Instant oatmeal **-1** with brown sugar **-1** | −2 | » Old-fashioned oatmeal **2** with sliced strawberries **2** and almond slivers **2** | 6 |
| **MORNING SNACK** | » Caramel nut brownie Luna bar **-2** | −2 | » Green superfood bar (berry) **1** | 1 |
| **LUNCH** | » Sandwich on enriched wheat bread **-1** with turkey **2**, cheese **1**, and mayo **-1** <br> » Potato chips **-2** <br> » Diet soda **-2** | −3 | » Sandwich on whole wheat bread **2**, with turkey **2**, cheese **2**, guacamole, lettuce, and cucumber **1** <br> » Carrot sticks **2** with ranch dressing **-1** <br> » V-8 **2** | 10 |
| **AFTERNOON SNACK** | » Yoplait fat-free yogurt **1** (strawberry cheesecake) **-2** | −1 | » Plain yogurt **1** with fresh blueberries **2** | 3 |
| **DINNER** | » Chicken breast **2** <br> » Couscous **-1** <br> » Green Giant frozen broccoli **2** with cheese sauce **-2** | 1 | » Chicken breast **2** <br> » Brown rice pilaf **2** <br> » Steamed broccoli **2** | 6 |
| **DESSERT** | » Chocolate ice cream **-2** | −2 | » Dark chocolate **0** | 0 |
| **DAILY TOTAL** | | −9 | | 26 |

simple ways to improve the quality of common types of meals and snacks eaten throughout the day.

The next way to improve your DQS is to add high-quality foods. I recommend that you add fruits and vegetables first, as these are the high-quality foods your diet most likely lacks. Add servings until you are consuming at least three and preferably four servings of each. Easy ways to add fruits and vegetables to your diet include adding fruits as mid-morning and midafternoon snacks and simply doubling vegetable portion sizes at meals. Don't be concerned that adding high-quality foods to your diet will promote weight gain. These foods provide more satiety than they do calories, so when you add them, you will naturally eat slightly less of other stuff.

There are different strategies you can use to improve your diet quality. If change is not difficult for you, it might be best for you to make a bunch of changes simultaneously. Other personalities might find it more effective to make one or two changes at a time. Naturally, the first approach will give you faster results, whereas the second is likely to feel less disruptive and overwhelming. Neither option is inherently better than the other, but each is better for some people. Consider your psychological makeup, and choose the option that will work best for you. Regardless of how you decide to begin improving your diet quality, be sure to calculate your daily DQS as long as the process of improving your diet lasts so that you can quantify your improvement and create a new personal target score.

The maximum possible score on the DQS is 32. You will achieve this score by eating four servings of fruits and vegetables and three servings of lean meats and fish, whole grains, nuts and seeds, and dairy and by not eating any low-quality foods whatsoever. You don't need to hit a DQS of 29 every day—or ever, for that matter—to reach your racing weight and maximize your endurance performance and overall health. Instead of trying to achieve a perfect DQS, focus instead on improving your existing score until you are satisfied with the results you get. Once you have arrived at that point, there is no need to improve it any further. Continue to calculate your DQS every once in a while to make sure you are hitting your personal target, whatever it is.

Table 4.3 presents three sample one-day food journals and their scores. The first is a very-low-quality day's eating that is unlikely to allow any athlete who eats it to attain his or her optimal racing weight,

TABLE 4.3 **SAMPLE DQS FOOD JOURNALS**

| FOOD JOURNAL 1 LOW QUALITY | FOOD JOURNAL 2 FAIRLY HIGH QUALITY | FOOD JOURNAL 3 HIGH QUALITY |
|---|---|---|
| » Kellogg's Froot Loops -2 | » Scrambled egg 2 | » Fruit and vegetable smoothie (orange juice, banana, strawberries, spinach 8 ) |
| » Skim milk 1 | » Whole wheat toast 2 with butter -1 | |
| » Starbuck's grande mocha latte -1 | » Orange juice 2 | » Plain yogurt 1 with fresh raspberries 1 |
| » M&M's -2 | » Banana 2 | |
| » Carne asada burrito (carne asada -1, white rice -1, pinto beans 2, and cheese 1) | » Chicken Caesar salad wrap -1 (chicken 2, veggies 2, dressing -1) | » Leftover chicken 2 and vegetable stir-fry 2 with brown rice 2 |
| » Diet soda -2 | » Sun Chips -2 | » Pear 1 |
| » Slim Jim -1 | » Apple juice 2 | » Marinated broiled haddock 2 |
| » Cheeseburger -2 | » Roasted cashews 2 | |
| » French fries -2 | » Spaghetti -1 with meatballs -2, and red sauce 2 | » Brown rice pilaf 2 |
| » Beer 0 | | » Steamed french beans 2 |
| » Frozen yogurt -2 | » Garden salad 2 | » Wine 0 |
| | » Iced green tea (unsweetened) 0 | » Dark chocolate 0 |
| **-12** | **12** | **23** |

assuming that portions are determined by appetite (which in turn is influenced primarily by body size and activity level). The second food journal represents a fairly high-quality day's eating that is likely to be sufficient for the attainment of optimal racing weight for some athletes but not others (again assuming that appetite determines the amount of food eaten). The third food journal represents a very-high-quality day's eating that is likely to facilitate optimal racing weight attainment in any athlete.

# FIVE

STEP 2

# MANAGING YOUR APPETITE

Throughout his career as a professional triathlete, Peter Reid worried constantly about his weight and worked hard to attain his racing weight for big events. The 6-foot-3-inch Canadian's "natural" weight—that is, the weight his body settled at when he ate healthily and trained consistently but took no additional weight-management measures—was 172 to 175 pounds. Experience taught Reid that he raced best at 164 to 165 pounds. His ability to reach this lower weight by controlling the amount of food he ate—in addition to eating healthily and training consistently—enabled him to win three Ironman World Championship titles between 1998 and 2003.

At the height of his training for Ironman each year, Reid emptied his refrigerator and pantry of food. His kitchen remained empty until he returned from Hawaii for the off-season. He shopped individually for every single meal he ate, brought the ingredients home, prepared them, and ate everything. When the meal was done, there was again not a crumb in the house to nibble on.

While Reid bought enough food to fuel as much as 35 hours a week of training, he did not buy enough to satisfy his hunger. This is precisely why he kept his pantry bare. He became so hungry between meals that no amount of willpower could have restrained him from eating whatever was available. When he went to bed, his hunger was sometimes so intense that it gave him a headache.

Reid recognized that his approach to weight management was not entirely healthy. "I know I have an issue with that," he said at the tail end of his career in 2005. "I have somewhat of an eating disorder."

While I won't deny that Reid's methods worked for him, I don't believe that any other endurance athlete needs to keep his kitchen food free or go to bed with a hunger headache to attain his racing weight. There was an underlying wisdom in Reid's efforts to regulate the amount of food he ate, however. He understood that relying entirely on willpower to avoid eating too much to attain racing weight is a mistake. The desire to eat is too strong to be overcome by mere self-restraint. Creating a personal environment and lifestyle that discourage overeating is also necessary. It is not enough to resist temptations; they must also be removed to some degree.

Science has substantiated the truth that Peter Reid intuited. Research on the physiology, psychology, and sociology of appetite and eating behavior has clearly demonstrated that most people have to do more than eat healthy foods and exercise to reach their ideal weight. They must also control the amount of food they eat because in the absence of such regulatory efforts, they eat too much food to achieve their goals for body composition.

Endurance athletes are no exception, and that's why managing your appetite is the second step of the Racing Weight system. Appetite management is not a matter of going hungry for the sake of getting leaner. It's about understanding how appetite works, recognizing the factors that influence how much food you eat, and exploiting this knowledge to reduce the number of calories you eat with minimal reliance on willpower, which can be a flimsy thing.

## MANAGING APPETITE VERSUS COUNTING CALORIES

The traditional method of regulating food intake is counting calories. Appetite management, in contrast, is a fundamentally different way of preventing overeating. With calorie counting you control the amount of food you eat by conscious thought, whereas with appetite management you control the amount of food you eat by feel plus a little manipulation of your "food environment" to make your feel for how much to eat more trustworthy.

Calorie counting is very sensible in principle. Losing weight requires that you eat fewer calories than your body uses. Counting calories helps you determine if you are in fact using more calories than you eat. Pretty simple.

## APPETITE MANAGEMENT IS A FUNDAMENTALLY DIFFERENT WAY OF PREVENTING OVEREATING.

But what's simple in principle can be difficult in practice. Counting calories is challenging for two reasons. First, it's a pain, requiring more time and effort than most people feel it is worth. There are actually two calculations involved. Before you start counting calories in foods, you must determine the number of calories your body burns each day. This is not easy, especially if you exercise a lot. The foundation of your total daily caloric expenditure is your basal metabolic rate, or the number of calories your body burns at rest in 24 hours. The second layer of your total daily caloric expenditure is the additional calories you burn through nonexercise activities. Your body uses calories at a slightly higher rate when you're driving a vehicle or working at a desk than when you're lying in bed, so these activities must be factored into your tally. Finally, your workouts need to be accounted for as well. This wouldn't be so hard if you did the same workout every day, but if your workouts vary from day to day, then each day requires a separate calculation.

Once you've established how many calories your body uses in a day, you are ready to start counting the calories in the foods you eat. If you're trying to maintain your current weight, you'll want to consume the same number of calories your body uses. If you're trying to lose weight, you'll want to consume slightly less. As anyone who has ever tried it knows, counting food calories is a bit of a hassle. It's easy enough if you eat all of your meals at restaurants that print the calorie count of every entrée, appetizer, and side item right on the menu, but it's much more difficult at home and elsewhere.

Suppose you make a beef and vegetable stew at home. To get an accurate calorie count for one serving of this meal, you'll need to look up the calorie information of each of its dozen or more ingredients and measure the amount you eat. It can be done—Lance Armstrong went through the trouble of measuring and weighing meals to get calorie counts throughout his cycling career—but most health-conscious eaters deem the process too great a hassle and skip the math.

The second problem with do-it-yourself methods of calorie counting is that they are not very accurate. Official calorie information provided on product labels and restaurant menus is not always reliable. In a 2011 study researchers at Tufts University found that 20 percent of 269 restaurant menu items that were tested contained significantly less or (more often) significantly more calories than they were supposed to have (Urban et al. 2011). Only 7 percent of the official calorie counts were within 10 calories of the actual number.

In an interview for *U.S. News and World Report* the study's lead author, Jean Mayer, stated, "I have a Ph.D. in nutrition, and I can't tell if my dinner is 500 or 800 calories just by looking at the plate, and our study shows you can't rely on the restaurants' numbers for an individual meal" (Haupt 2011).

Even if you are willing to endure the hassle of counting calories, your calculations could easily be 10 percent inaccurate or more. Instead of eating 5 percent fewer calories than your body uses and losing weight, you might consume 5 percent more and gain weight. It's true that people who do count calories seldom overeat because the process makes them more mindful of their eating. But there's an easier way to eat mindfully: appetite management.

Wild animals are incapable of counting calories, yet they rarely overeat. For that matter, human beings lacked any concept of calories until the late 19th century, yet it was only after calorie counting became possible that overeating became a widespread problem for our species. How do wild animals control the amount of food they eat? They do it by listening to their bodies and by relying on a food environment in which overeating would be difficult even if their body signals were unreliable. How did human beings before the rise of the obesity epidemic in the 1970s control the amount of food they ate? By the same means.

For better or worse, we cannot go backward in time. The modern human food environment makes overeating all too easy, and even though there may be a way forward (think of recent municipal bans on sales of oversized soft drinks), for now we're stuck. It is possible, however, to change your personal food environment to make it easier to avoid overeating, as Peter Reid did with his empty kitchen. It is also possible to rediscover how to rely on your own body signals as a means of properly regulating food intake. Appetite management in the Racing Weight system is a collection of methods for creating a better personal food environment and eating mindfully.

# WHY WE OVEREAT

Appetite—which we can define simply as the desire to eat—is a complex phenomenon. There is no tidy answer to the question, Why do people eat as much as they do? Physiological, psychological, and sociological factors are involved.

Most people think that declining blood glucose levels are the primary physiological stimulus for hunger, but the link between blood glucose and hunger is in fact relatively weak. A link does exist, however. When the blood glucose level falls, regions of the brain that help us resist food temptations are weakened. So you see that the physiological and psychological dimensions of appetite are not really separate.

A much more potent hunger trigger than low blood glucose is an empty stomach. When the stomach is empty, certain hunger-causing hormones are released. The most powerful hunger hormone is ghrelin, which the stomach secretes when it is empty. Human subjects who are injected with ghrelin become ravenous even when their stomachs are full. A rare genetic disorder known as Prater-Willi syndrome causes chronically high circulating ghrelin levels and constant, uncontrollable hunger.

Even ghrelin is influenced by psychological factors. Ghrelin is known to function on a circadian schedule, generating hunger at the same times every day. But this schedule is adaptable, so if you change your eating schedule, your "hunger schedule" will quickly adjust (LeSauter et al. 2009). Think of it as a form of Pavlovian conditioning.

Scientists draw a distinction between physical hunger and hedonic hunger. Appetite, or the desire to eat, encompasses both. Physical hunger (or "belly hunger" as I like to call it) is a set of signals, including a rumbling stomach, that communicates a real need for food from the body to the mind. Hedonic hunger (or "head hunger") is the desire to eat for pleasure. You might think that a hormone such as ghrelin would underlie belly hunger but not head hunger. This is not the case.

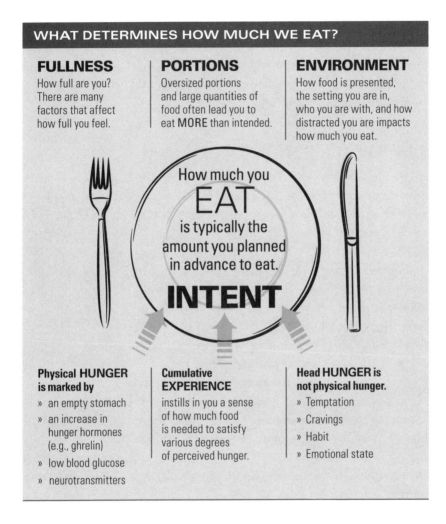

## WHAT DETERMINES HOW MUCH WE EAT?

**FULLNESS**
How full are you?
There are many
factors that affect
how full you feel.

**PORTIONS**
Oversized portions
and large quantities of
food often lead you to
eat MORE than intended.

**ENVIRONMENT**
How food is presented,
the setting you are in,
who you are with, and how
distracted you are impacts
how much you eat.

How much you
EAT
is typically the
amount you planned
in advance to eat.
INTENT

**Physical HUNGER
is marked by**
» an empty stomach
» an increase in
  hunger hormones
  (e.g., ghrelin)
» low blood glucose
» neurotransmitters

**Cumulative
EXPERIENCE**
instills in you a sense
of how much food
is needed to satisfy
various degrees
of perceived hunger.

**Head HUNGER is
not physical hunger.**
» Temptation
» Cravings
» Habit
» Emotional state

In a 2012 study Italian researchers showed that food temptations experienced in the absence of physical hunger stimulate ghrelin, just as an empty stomach does (Monteleone et al. 2012). The experiment involved adult men and women who were healthy and not overweight. The subjects were fed a standardized breakfast and then asked to rate their level of hunger. An hour later, each subject was presented with his or her favorite food and asked to reassess his or her hunger level. On a separate occasion the experiment was repeated, but in this case the subjects were presented with a food that they did not like.

The subjects reported experiencing a sudden spike in hunger when they were presented with their favorite food just one hour after a satisfying breakfast. When presented with an unappetizing food in the same circumstance, however, there was no increase in appetite. What's more, blood samples revealed that there was also a spike in ghrelin (a hunger hormone) when the favorite food was displayed—a spike that did not occur in the presence of the unappetizing food.

Hormones also play a role in determining when we stop eating after we've started. One of the major satiety hormones is cholecystokinin (CCK). CCK is secreted by the small intestine when the presence of fat from a meal is detected. The hormone then slows the movement of food through the intestinal tract so that it can be properly digested and sends a signal to the brain that diminishes the desire to eat.

There are many degrees of fullness. People seldom eat until they are so full they can't eat another bite. But there is no clear fullness threshold below this limit at which people stop eating every time they eat. Of course, almost everyone habitually eats to a level of fullness that ensures the body gets enough energy to maintain health. But there is a lot of room between the thresholds of eating enough to barely keep hunger at an acceptable level and eating to the point of uncomfortable fullness. The exact degree of fullness that is felt at the cessation of eating varies from person to person and from meal to meal. There is evidence that psychological factors such as the taste of the food being eaten and the amount of variety in the meal affect how much is eaten. The more variety there is on the plate, the more we eat.

Perhaps the most powerful psychological determinant of how much we eat and how full we get is intent. People usually plan how much they are going to eat before they start and then eat that amount, regardless of how full it makes them. For example, a person orders a particular entrée at a restaurant and eats the whole thing, neither stopping four bites shy of clearing the plate because he feels full enough nor ordering a second entrée and eating only four bites because the first plate leaves him not quite full enough.

Naturally, our eating plans are not arbitrary. The amounts of food we plan to eat in meals are shaped by experience. We have a sense of how much is enough in various circumstances, so we habitually plan to eat those amounts. This is where the sociological dimension of appetite enters the picture. Our habitual portion sizes are largely determined by social forces rather than by individual inclination. In other words, we tend to eat the amounts that those around us eat. From the time we are preschoolers, we are trained how much to eat by restaurant serving sizes, packaged food portions, and even the sizes of the plates and bowls we eat from and the glasses we drink from. We trust that the amounts we are offered are normal, and we consume these amounts regardless of what our body signals try to tell us.

## THE MOST POWERFUL PSYCHOLOGICAL DETERMINANT OF HOW MUCH WE EAT AND HOW FULL WE GET IS INTENT.

Between the time we are born and age 3, we rely on internal signals almost exclusively to determine how much we eat. But at age 3 we begin to rely on external cues and ignore internal signals. When researchers from Penn State University and Baylor Medical School fed either medium or large portions of macaroni and cheese to three-year-olds, the children ate roughly the same amount despite the difference in the amount of food offered (Fisher, Rolls, and Birch 2003). The experiment was then repeated with five-year-olds, who ate 26 percent more when they were given large servings.

Interestingly, there appears to be some variability in the degree to which older children and adults rely on social influences versus internal cues in different cultures. A study conducted by Brian Wansink, author of *Mindless Eating*, found that Americans tended to stop eating when they simply ran out of food on their plate, whereas the French tended to stop when they felt full, regardless of whether there was food left on their plate (Wansink, Payne, and Chandon 2007). The bad news here is that the American food environment facilitates overeating more than other cultural food environments do. The good news is that the French prove it is possible to eat by the body's dictates even as an adult.

There are really two reasons that many people in wealthy societies generally, and Americans in particular, overeat. One problem is that a lot of the most commonly eaten foods in the modern diet have much greater caloric density than the foods our ancestors ate when our appetite control mechanisms evolved. Those mechanisms were designed to work with natural, unprocessed foods—most of which have relatively low calorie density—to ensure that we eat neither too little nor too much.

Some of the factors that influence how much we eat depend on lower caloric densities to function appropriately. These factors include the amount of chewing that is done, the amount of time we spend eating, and the volume of the food we intend to eat (or how big it looks). When you eat a calorically dense modern food such as a cheeseburger, you may easily consume more calories than you need without eating a volume of food that appears to be too much and without doing an unacceptable amount of chewing or spending a burdensome amount of time eating. This is much less likely with an unprocessed natural food such as a spinach salad or even a piece of fish.

An Ultimate Cheeseburger from Jack in the Box contains 819 calories, or about a third of the calories the average runner needs in an entire day. This sandwich can be eaten in three minutes without haste. A filet of codfish that is equal to the Ultimate Cheeseburger in weight contains fewer than 200 calories. A person is very unlikely to serve himself 819 calories' worth of codfish, which would appear to be way too much on a plate, or to chew 819 calories' worth of codfish.

Because unnaturally calorie-dense foods are one of the two major causes of overeating, limiting these foods in favor of natural, unprocessed foods is one of the most effective ways to avoid overeating. You're already doing this by following step 1 of the Racing Weight system— improving your diet quality. But there are other ways to avoid overeating that address the second cause of overeating: today's fattening food environment.

As I've mentioned, people usually eat the amount of food they plan to eat, and the amount they habitually plan to eat is influenced by a sense of "normal" portion sizes that is culturally established. If a single-serving bag of potato chips contain 1.5 ounces of food, most people will eat one full bag. If a single-serving bag of potato chips contain 2 ounces of food (or about 80 more calories than a 1.5-ounce bag), most people will still eat one full bag.

Portion sizes in America increased drastically between the start of the obesity epidemic in the 1970s and its peak in the first decade of the 21st century. The trend started in restaurants and with packaged supermarket foods. Advancements in industrial food production methods caused the cost of food to plummet, creating competition between restaurants and food manufacturers to compete for customers on the basis of providing value, or more food for less money. According to a study conducted by the Centers for Disease Control and Prevention, the average fast-food restaurant portion size *quadrupled* between the 1950s and early 2000s (Young and Nestle 2007). Over that same span of time the average American adult became 26 pounds heavier.

> **MANY PEOPLE IN WEALTHY SOCIETIES GENERALLY, AND AMERICANS IN PARTICULAR, OVEREAT.**

Research has also shown that portion sizes served at home increased in parallel with those offered at restaurants and in packaged foods. People were trained by the food industry to consider larger portions normal and behaved accordingly even when eating meals made from scratch in the kitchen (Popkin and Nielsen 2003).

It can be discouraging to realize how much of our eating behavior is controlled by our environment. But this very awareness creates an opportunity to exercise greater self-determination for the sake of avoiding excessive eating. There are many ways you can use your knowledge of how your appetite works to manage it and move a step closer to your Racing Weight, none of which needs to be as extreme as Peter Reid's methods.

## HOW NOT TO OVEREAT

There are eight especially effective ways of managing appetite. You may not need to use all of them to attain your racing weight, but I recommend that every endurance athlete practice at least the first of these measures.

### 1. LEARN THE DIFFERENCE BETWEEN BELLY HUNGER AND HEAD HUNGER.

In 2008 a team of researchers led by Mario Ciampolini of the University of Firenze studied the effects on body weight of training overweight persons to eat whenever and only when they experienced belly hunger (Ciampolini, Lovell-Smith, and Sifone 2010). In the first seven weeks of the five-month study, volunteers were trained to distinguish belly hunger from head hunger. The main symptoms of belly hunger were gastric pangs, feelings of emptiness or hollowness, and mental and physical weakness. The subjects were instructed to eat within an hour of noticing these symptoms and to not eat again until they returned. They were also encouraged to adjust the types and amounts of food they ate in meals as well as their timing so that belly hunger tended to arise on a predictable timetable that allowed them to maintain a consistent eating schedule.

The volunteers were allowed to eat whatever they wanted. They were also allowed to eat as much as they wanted at each meal as long as they were not still full when it was time for their next meal. If symptoms of belly hunger did not return before the next scheduled meal, they knew they had eaten too much and should eat a little less in the next day's corresponding meal.

This one change in the eating patterns of the overweight subjects included in this study—elimination of eating for head hunger—yielded an average weight loss of nearly 15 pounds in five months. That shows you how much "mindless eating" we are inclined to do if left to our own discretion.

The most powerful thing you can do to lose excess body fat through appetite management is to re-create this experiment in your own life. I recommend that you start by choosing a weekend (weekends are better because of the freedom they afford to dispose of time as you please) on which to abandon your normal eating schedule and eat only when you experience symptoms of belly hunger: gastric pangs, feelings of emptiness or hollowness, and mental or physical weakness. Eat a normal meal within an hour of the emergence of these symptoms, and then wait until they reappear to eat your next meal. Do not eat when you simply feel like eating and do not have symptoms of belly hunger. Continue doing this for two full days.

The purpose of this test is to learn the difference between belly hunger and head hunger and get used to resisting head hunger and eating only when belly hunger is present. On Monday go back to your normal eating schedule, but try to adjust the amounts you eat so that you experience symptoms of belly hunger before it's time to eat again (but not more than an hour before it's time to eat again). If you find this difficult, you'll probably have to change your habitual eating schedule (although changing the content of your meals may also do the trick in some circumstances).

For example, suppose you normally eat a snack at 3:00 in the afternoon, but after beginning to practice this method of appetite management, you discover that you cannot eat this snack and still experience belly hunger before your normal 6:00 dinner. In this case you'll need to eliminate that snack or perhaps push your dinner back to 7:00.

When I changed my diet in this way, I made no major changes to my eating schedule, but I started eating 10 to 20 percent less in most meals because that's what it took to ensure I was hungry again before my next meal. Although I had to get used to resisting a second-nature impulse to stuff myself and avoiding spontaneous food temptations, such as walking through my kitchen just as my wife removed a tray of fresh-baked muffins from the oven, it wasn't very hard because, after all, I was always allowed to eat when I was truly hungry. I think that you will find this method of appetite management equally eye-opening, easy, and effective.

Like all dietary "rules," this one should not be absolute. It's okay once in a while to eat a treat spontaneously when you're not truly hungry.

**2. CLEAN OUT YOUR KITCHEN.** While I advise you not to copy Peter Reid's example of completely emptying the kitchen of all foods, I do recommend that you go through your refrigerator and pantry and remove most or all of the low-quality temptations you find. You will be much less likely to eat low-quality indulgences if doing so is inconvenient, requiring a trip to the store.

Fortunately, people's laziness is even more powerful than their desire for high-calorie foods. In another of Brian Wansink's studies, secretaries were given a free dish of chocolates that was "magically" refilled at the end of every workday. One week the dish was positioned on a corner of their desk. Another week it was placed inside one of their desk drawers. A third week the dish was placed six feet away from their desks. On average the secretaries ate nine chocolates a day when the chocolates were most conveniently located, six a day when they were out of sight but close by, and only four a day when the treats were least conveniently located (Painter, Wansink, and Hieggelke 2002).

Keeping a "clean kitchen" exploits our laziness in order to make appetite management easy. Once your kitchen is clean, keep it clean by no longer buying low-quality treats at the supermarket to take home. If you're like me, you'll find that it's a lot easier to resist treats that you would not eat immediately even if you did buy them than it is to resist those same treats once they're already in your home.

Naturally, the more you eat at home instead of at restaurants, the more you benefit from keeping a clean kitchen.

**3. USE SMALLER DISHES**. As portion sizes have increased over the past several decades, so has the size of the plates and bowls we eat from at home. If you ever see a 100-year-old dinner plate, you'll probably think it's a salad plate. Research has shown that people naturally eat smaller portions when they eat from smaller dishes. What's more, they don't feel less satisfied, because it's still possible to eat enough to cover belly hunger from antique-size dishes, whereas today's dishes encourage overeating.

Donate your dishes to Goodwill or the Salvation Army, and shop for an attractive new set of smaller sizes. Once you have them, you will automatically pour and eat smaller bowls of breakfast cereal and serve and eat smaller helpings of lasagna. This is another appetite management method that is most effective when you eat most of your meals at home.

**4. SPOIL YOUR APPETITE**. You may find it easier to avoid overeating at meals if you start each meal by filling some space in your stomach with a food or liquid that has low calorie density. You can make this method as simple as drinking a large glass of whatever before you sit down to eat. A study led by Brenda Davy at Virginia Tech University reported that subjects ate 75 to 90 fewer calories in meals that were preceded by the swallowing of 16 ounces of water (Dennis et al. 2010). Earlier research by Barbara Rolls determined that broth-based soup had a similar effect when consumed before solid food (Flood and Rolls 2007).

If you're having a salad instead of soup with your meal, try eating the entire salad before you eat anything else. Like water and soup, a salad appetizer will put you well on the way toward satiety without a lot of calories.

**5. KEEP HEALTHY FOODS HANDY**. In addition to making it less convenient to eat low-quality foods at home, make it more convenient to eat high-quality foods away from home. If you keep healthy foods with low calorie density close at hand, you will be less likely to overeat unhealthy foods with high calorie density when belly hunger sneaks up on you at the office, on the road, and elsewhere.

Stash fresh or dried fruit, nuts, or jerky in your desk at the office. Keep a few real-food snack bars in your car and your airplane carry-on bag. Remember, people are lazy. If healthy snacks are always within reach, you will use them to manage your appetite instead of going for the usual conveniences of vending machines and fast-food drive-thru windows.

**6. PLAN FOR TEMPTATION.** Many opportunities to eat for head hunger take us by surprise. Recently I went to the local farmer's market to buy some fresh organic fruits and vegetables with my wife. As we strolled along, a man who was handing out free kettle corn to attract customers to his kettle corn booth approached me, and before I knew it my hands were full of the stuff, which I dutifully ate.

Psychologists recommend the use of a technique called "implementation intention" to handle such situations. This is the practice of making specific plans for dealing with temptations before they arise. For example, I might have created an intention to politely request "just a taste" of the next free treat I was offered by surprise in public. With such a plan in place, I would have been less likely to eat the two handfuls of kettle corn I ate at the farmer's market.

Implementation intentions can be specific to situations. For example, "If Aunt Margie offers me brownies when I visit, as she usually does, I will tell her I just ate and ask if I can take a few home. On the way home, I will give them to that hungry-looking guy I always see on the corner of Elm and 4th." Implementation intentions can also be framed broadly so that they cover some of the least expected temptations. For example, "Anytime I am tempted to have a second drink—be it wine, beer, or spirits, at home or away from home, alone or in the company of others—I will have a breath mint instead."

> ❞ THE KEY TO AVOIDING THE COMMON PROBLEM OF OVEREATING IS SIMPLE AWARENESS.

One of the most common causes of head hunger eating (and drinking) is what I call the "just this once" delusion. When a surprise chance to indulge comes about, we tell ourselves that we will give in to the temptation just this once and then resist all future temptations. The problem is that when the next opportunity comes, we've already forgotten about the last indulgence, and we're able to tell ourselves "just this once" again. Implementation intentions pull the rug out from under this delusion.

**7. AVOID DISTRACTED EATING.** Much of the eating we do today is distracted eating—eating in front of television and computer screens and behind steering wheels. Research has shown that people tend to eat more when distracted because they are even less attuned to their body signals than normal. Listening to music during meals and even eating with other people increase food intake (Stroebele and Castro 2004).

Totally distraction-free eating is not realistic or desirable for most of us. Who wants to eat every meal alone in silence? But if distracted eating is a major source of head hunger eating in your life, you may need to eliminate certain distractions. Even establishing a single rule that forbids you from eating while watching television could make a difference.

**8. LIMIT VARIETY.** We don't overeat at buffets only because buffets offer all you can eat. We also overeat because there's so much to choose from. We automatically eat more when we have more flavors, textures, and even colors to sample in a meal. Followers of diets such as the Paleo Diet often believe that the key to their effectiveness is the elimination of "bad" foods. Many experts believe that these diets actually yield results because they reduce dietary variety.

If you have a lunch comprising a sandwich, soup, and a salad, you will probably eat more than you would if you ate only a sandwich and a salad, even if you intended to eat smaller amounts of the meal with less variety. Reducing the variety of foods in meals can be an effective way to eat less for those who tend to take a buffet-style approach to their meals. Naturally, you don't want to eliminate so much variety that your diet quality suffers. But you can have it both ways by making meals of single foods that incorporate nutritional variety, such as a chicken and vegetable stir-fry over brown rice, which your brain will interpret as a single food because every bite is more or less the same.

# EATING WITH INTENTION

In a 2009 study researchers at the University of Washington found that men and women who regularly practiced yoga were significantly thinner than people who practiced other forms of exercise (Framson et al. 2009). The reason had to do with another finding of the study, which was that yoga participants scored significantly higher on a standard mindful eating questionnaire. The authors of the study speculated that yoga, which trains people in body awareness, gave its regular participants a better sense of their real food needs, resulting in less eating and lower body weight.

The lesson here for endurance athletes is not that we should all take up yoga. Rather, it is that the key to avoiding the common problem of overeating is simple awareness. You don't have to count calories or go hungry to guarantee that you take in enough calories each day and no more. You just have to pay attention to your body and learn the difference between belly hunger and head hunger; notice your thoughts, emotions, and environment to discover your greatest personal vulnerabilities to overeating; and make a few simple changes to your routines that ensure you always eat intentionally.

# SIX

# STEP 3

# BALANCING
# YOUR ENERGY SOURCES

Haile Gebrselassie is widely considered to be history's greatest runner. It would be difficult indeed to argue that any other runner has achieved more than the Ethiopian great's two Olympic gold medals, eight world championship gold medals, and 27 world records. His range—from 3:31.76 (indoors) for 1,500 meters to 2:03:59 for the marathon—is certainly unmatched. So is his longevity. In 1992 Gebrselassie won gold medals at 5,000 and 10,000 meters at the World Junior Championships in Athletics. Twenty years later he won the highly competitive Great Manchester run (a 10K) with a time of 27:39.

One of the keys to Gebrselassie's spectacularly prolonged success was a consistent routine that he once described as "breakfast, running, lunch, running, dinner." A highly successful businessman and active civic leader, Geb actually squeezed a good deal of work between his runs and meals, but he never gave training short shrift or compromised the quality of his diet.

His typical breakfast consisted of several pieces of bread with butter and jam, orange juice, and tea with sugar. Lunch is traditionally the biggest meal of the day for Ethiopians, and so it usually was for Gebrselassie. Most days he ate *injera*, a spongy bread made with whole-grain teff, which he used to wrap cooked vegetables and traditional Ethiopian meat preparations, such as *doro wat,* a spicy chicken dish. He washed these foods down with more tea and perhaps also a small cup of Ethiopian coffee or *tege,* a mildly alcoholic drink made from honey and barley.

At the dinner table Geb favored pastas, such as spaghetti and macaroni. While pasta is not a traditional Ethiopian dish, it has been quite popular there since the Italians tried to colonize the country in the 1940s. A well-traveled man, "The Emperor" enjoys many Western foods, including fast food, but he only allowed himself to eat that after victories.

ETHIOPIAN RUNNERS CONSUMED NEARLY

**10** GRAMS

**OF CARBS**
*per kilogram of body weight daily.*

Even more striking than the overall quality of the diet of history's greatest runner was its extremely high carbohydrate content. Almost everything he ate and drank in a typical day, aside from a little lean meat, was carb-rich. In this respect Gebrselassie's diet was not unlike that of other Ethiopian runners. An analysis of the diets of 10 world-class Ethiopian runners conducted in 2011 by a team of European and Ethiopian researchers determined that on average these athletes consumed nearly 10 grams of carbs per kilogram of body weight daily, or about 2.5 times the amount of carbs (adjusted for body weight) that the typical American eats (Beis et al. 2011).

There are some sports nutrition authorities who believe that no athlete should get more than 40 to 50 percent of his calories from carbs. If they are correct, then the East African runners eat far too much carbohydrate. That's an absurd idea. East Africa's runners are by far the best in the world. Remember, the dietary habits and training methods of the world's best endurance athletes define what works. These athletes hold most of the records, they win most of the big races, and they eat a lot of carbohydrates. We need no other proof that a high-carbohydrate diet is good for hard-training endurance athletes.

Yet there is other proof. A number of studies have demonstrated that endurance athletes are able to train harder and perform better in hard training when they eat a lot of carbs. In fact, scientific evidence suggests that many endurance athletes in Western countries don't consume enough carbohydrates to support their training loads optimally. So why does a vocal minority in the endurance sports community—including proponents of the Zone Diet and the Paleo Diet—believe that a low-carbohydrate diet is best for endurance athletes?

Anticarb sentiment in the endurance sports community is an ideological spillover from the weight-loss diet culture. Low-carb diets for weight loss have been popular for many years. These diets are based on the idea that carbohydrates are responsible for weight gain and on its logical corollary: that cutting carbs is the most effective way to lose weight. Advocates of low-carb diets for endurance athletes believe that the same principles apply to those who train hard every day, but they also believe that low-carb diets are better for endurance performance because they train the muscles to burn fat more effectively, which in turn boosts fatigue resistance.

In fact, carbohydrate consumption per se is not responsible for weight gain in the general population. While cutting carbs from the diet can be an effective way to lose weight, it is no more effective than other dietary approaches to weight loss. So for nonathletes the decision to use a low-carb diet for weight loss is a matter of personal preference. But for endurance athletes low-carb diets are not the best way to get leaner because, as I've suggested, they compromise training capacity. High-carb diets increase training capacity and enhance training performance, and these effects in turn tend to improve body composition. Remember, anything you do as an athlete that helps you perform better is likely to make you leaner as well; including enough carbohydrates in your diet is another example of this principle.

## HIGH-CARB DIETS INCREASE TRAINING CAPACITY AND ENHANCE TRAINING PERFORMANCE—EFFECTS THAT IN TURN IMPROVE BODY COMPOSITION.

All three of the energy sources, or macronutrients, in the diet—carbohydrate, fat, and protein—are important. But for the endurance athlete carbohydrate is most important because carbohydrate needs increase drastically as training increases, whereas fat and protein needs increase more moderately. Failure to get enough of any macronutrient will hurt your training, but few endurance athletes fail to get enough fat or protein, whereas inadequate carbohydrate intake is common. Of course, getting enough carbohydrate matters little if your diet quality is low, you manage your appetite poorly, and you don't follow the other steps of the Racing Weight plan. But real-world and scientific evidence suggest that if you do adhere to the other steps, you will perform better and get leaner on a high-carb diet than you will on a carb-restricted diet for athletes such as the Zone Diet or the Paleo Diet.

# LOW-CARB WEIGHT-LOSS DIETS

One of the earliest champions of the idea that carbohydrate was the chief culprit in weight gain was Alfred Pennington, a physician and researcher for the Du Pont chemical company in the 1940s. Pennington was led to this conclusion through his search for a diet that would yield weight loss "automatically" without consciously enforced calorie restriction. Evidence at the time suggested that pyruvic acid, which the body produces through carbohydrate metabolism, was responsible for excess fat storage. Pennington hypothesized that a reduction of carbohydrate in the diet would correspondingly reduce pyruvic acid production and fat storage even while the dieter continued to eat enough fat and protein to fully satisfy his or her appetite.

Pennington was aware that the body requires stable blood glucose levels for normal functioning and that carbohydrate restriction threatens blood glucose stability. But it had recently been shown that the body is able to maintain stable blood glucose levels despite carbohydrate restriction by breaking down stored body fat to produce glucose "substitutes" known as ketones. Thus, it seemed that low-carbohydrate diets offered a unique way of causing the body to aggressively break down its fat stores to meet its own energy needs.

Another advantage of low-carbohydrate diets for weight loss, Pennington noted, was that they did not cause the body's basal metabolic rate (or the rate of calorie burning at rest) to decline, whereas general calorie-restriction diets did. What more could a dieter have asked for? Current knowledge in human nutrition and metabolism indicated that low-carb diets would reduce fat storage, increase fat burning, allow unrestricted eating, and keep the body's metabolic rate from falling—a "perfect storm" of conditions for quick and easy weight loss. All Pennington needed was evidence that they actually worked.

Pennington got his proof when he devised a low-carb diet and tested it on Du Pont employees. The diet required that subjects eat at least 8 ounces of fatty meat three times a day along with a small portion of either white potatoes, sweet potatoes, rice, grapefruit, melon, banana, pear, raspberries, or blueberries. Almost everyone who tried the diet lost weight, and the 20 obese individuals who followed it lost an average of 22 pounds over a period of three-and-a-half months.

In 1963, some 10 years after Pennington published his findings, a young physician named Robert Atkins, who was himself overweight, read about them and was inspired. He tried a low-carb diet, lost weight, and then began to prescribe the diet to his patients. In a 1972 book about the "Atkins Nutritional Approach," Atkins expanded Pennington's original theory about why carbohydrates were fattening. He argued that high-carbohydrate diets caused the body to overproduce insulin, a hormone that plays a role in delivering excess carbs to adipose tissue for conversion into fat. Atkins also believed that eating too much carbohydrate caused large fluctuations in blood glucose and insulin levels, which in turn led to cravings for more carbohydrates and hence to overeating. Overweight persons were essentially addicted to carbohydrates, he said.

**THE WEIGHT LOSS THAT MANY PEOPLE EXPERIENCE ON LOW-CARB DIETS IS ATTRIBUTED TO REDUCED CALORIE INTAKE.**

By 2000 the Atkins Nutritional Approach had become the most popular weight-loss diet in history. Members of the nutrition science establishment, who preferred to blame dietary fat for making people fat, subjected low-carb diets to more rigorous scientific testing than they had been subjected to previously. If they hoped to prove that such diets were ineffective, those hopes were dashed. A study led by Will Yancy at the Duke University Medical Center found that obese individuals lost on average of 26 pounds in six months on the Atkins diet (McClernon et al. 2007). Another group of subjects placed on a low-fat diet lost only 14 pounds in an equal span of time.

Even as low-carb diets were validated as a means to lose weight, however, their theoretical underpinnings were dismantled by other research.

Careful studies revealed that the weight loss that resulted from low-carb diets had little to do with ketones, insulin, and cravings. The real reason people lost weight on the Atkins diet and other low-carb diets was that they ate fewer calories. Scientists were able to show that when calories were held equal, low-carb and low-fat diets yielded equal amounts of weight loss.

Low-carb diets might nevertheless be judged superior to other weight-loss diets if research could show that it was easier to eat fewer calories on them, but this evidence is lacking. After 10 years of intensive scientific comparisons of low-carb and other diets, the most that can be said for them is that they are about as effective as any other type of diet that reduces calorie intake.

And how effective is that? Not very effective in the real world. The true goal of any weight-loss diet is not short-term but permanent weight loss. Short-term weight loss is much easier to achieve. But only an esti-mated 20 percent of cases of significant short-term weight loss ultimately become permanent. The trouble with most studies of weight-loss diets is that their duration is short. Almost any reasonable dietary intervention will result in short-term weight loss that investigators can crow about in their published reports. But the few existing long-term studies have consistently shown that, regardless of what sort of diet is used, adher-ences drops after six months or so and subjects start to regain the weight they've lost. By two years after the diet began, the vast majority of dieters have regained all the weight they lost initially.

The only truly reliable proof of what works for permanent weight loss is data collected from people who have achieved such a loss on their own. Studies involving large groups of "successful" losers have found that no single particular type of diet is favored over any other. Some use low-fat diets, others use low-carb diets, still others rely on commercial plans such as Weight Watchers, and yet others make up their own rules. There is no pattern.

The real secrets to success in this population, research suggests, are behavioral factors such as self-monitoring (primarily through fre-quent weighing) and highly consistent eating patterns (Wing and Phelan 2005). The ratio of macronutrients in the diet is totally irrelevant to long-term weight-management outcomes. The effects of high-carb and low-carb diets on body weight in endurance athletes have not been stud-ied, but there is no reason to believe that low-carb diets are any more likely to yield permanent weight loss in endurance athletes than in non-athletes. A highly motivated endurance athlete could use a low-carb diet to get leaner, but not without risking a drop in training capacity and performance that would in turn limit his or her improvements in body composition.

## CARBOHYDRATE AND ENDURANCE PERFORMANCE

Unlike fat and protein, carbohydrate is not incorporated structurally into any body tissues. It is used only as fuel. Carbohydrate is stored in the liver and muscles as glycogen, but these stores are small—not even enough to fuel a marathon. This is why our carbohydrate needs are sensitive to our activity level. A desk worker who engages in no formal exercise needs very little carbohydrate and in fact shouldn't consume much carbohydrate because any excess is converted to fat for long-term storage in adipose tissue. But a serious endurance athlete may need two or even three times as much carbohydrate as the average person.

The importance of glycogen availability to exercise capacity and the known depleting effect of low-carbohydrate diets on glycogen stores caused some scientists to wonder if low-carb diets might hurt exercise capacity in weight-loss seekers on the Atkins Nutritional Approach and related diets. Studies involving overweight, sedentary individuals have found that their exercise capacity—which is low—is not made any lower by a low-carb diet. Even though glycogen stores are depleted by such a diet, subjects have been able to maintain their original (low) exercise capacity by relying more on fat to fuel exertion.

That's good news for overweight couch potatoes on low-carb diets who are contemplating starting an exercise program. These findings have little relevance to endurance athletes, however. Research going back to the 1960s has proven that the performance of trained athletes in racelike endurance tests is significantly affected by glycogen storage levels. When glycogen stores are maximized by a high-carbohydrate diet, endurance performance goes up. When glycogen stores are depleted by a low-carb diet, athletes bonk much sooner.

A serious **ENDURANCE ATHLETE** may need **2 or even 3 times as much carbohydrate** as the average person.

The discovery of this causal link by Swedish scientists inspired the practice of pre-race carbo-loading (Rowell, Masoro, and Spencer 1965).

Most endurance athletes carbo-load before races. But they often overlook the importance of keeping muscles well stocked with glycogen throughout the training process, when glycogen stores are being drawn on heavily day after day. Numerous studies have demonstrated that athletes who eat more carbohydrates are able to maintain a higher performance capacity during periods of heavy training.

One such study was performed by Asker Jeukendrup and his colleagues at the University of Birmingham, England, in 2004. A triathlete himself, Jeukendrup compared the effects of a high-carb diet (8.5 grams of carbohydrate per kilogram of body weight per day, or 65 percent of total calories) and a low-carb diet (5.4 grams of carbohydrate per kilogram per day, or 41 percent of total calories) on running performance during a period of intensified training. Seven high-level runners spent 11 days on each diet. Their training load was substantially increased for the last week of each 11-day period. At the beginning and again at the end of each heavy training period, the runners completed an 8-km time trial on the treadmill and a 16-km time trial outdoors. On both diets, the runners ran worse in the 8-km time trial after heavy training, but performance in the 16-km time trial worsened after heavy training only on the low-carb diet (Achten et al. 2004).

The more an athlete trains, the more carbohydrates that athlete needs in the diet to maintain performance. A good illustration of this principle is to be found in the diet of Greek ultrarunner Yiannis Kouros during a five-day, 600-mile race. To get through that event, Kouros had to eat and drink a tremendous number of calories—almost 12,000 per day—and nearly all of these calories—95.3 percent—came from carbohydrates. Kouros was wise to fuel his body in this seemingly unbalanced manner, as the body of a trained endurance athlete cannot store more than about 800 grams of carbohydrates (nonathletes store less than 400 grams) yet burns carbs at a rate of nearly 1 gram per minute even during moderate-intensity exercise such as ultrarunning. Thus, if Kouros had consumed "only" the 9.7 grams of carbohydrate

> The endurance athlete's body can store
>
> **800 g**
>
> **OF CARBOHYDRATES,**
> but it will
>
> **BURN CARBS**
> at a rate of
>
> **1 g/min.**
>
> of moderate exercise.

per kilogram of body weight that Ethiopian runners who run "only" 110 miles per week consume, his glycogen stores would have been depleted long before he reached the finish line (even though the body can convert a certain amount of dietary fat into carbohydrate).

## THE AMOUNT OF CARBOHYDRATE IN YOUR DAILY DIET SHOULD FLUCTUATE BASED ON YOUR TRAINING LOAD.

Most endurance athletes exercise a lot more than the overweight sedentary folks whose exercise capacity is not affected by low-carb eating and a lot less than Yiannis Kouros during his running stage race. Therefore, the carbohydrate needs of most endurance athletes also fall somewhere between these extremes. Studies in which the carbohydrate intake of moderately trained athletes has been manipulated have generally shown that the average American diet—which supplies a moderate 3 to 4 grams of carbohydrates per kilogram of body weight—maintains glycogen stores well enough to prevent a drop in performance. For example, a study by William Sherman at Ohio State University showed that runners and cyclists performed just as well in exhaustive exercise tests after seven days on a moderate-carbohydrate diet as they did after seven days on a high-carbohydrate diet, despite the fact that the moderate-carb diet reduced their muscle-glycogen stores by 30 to 36 percent compared to the high-carbohydrate diet (Sherman et al. 1993).

What lands athletes in trouble is switching to low-carbohydrate diets, such as the Zone Diet, that promise to increase endurance performance by boosting the fat-burning capacity of the muscle. Such diets do increase the muscles' reliance on fat for energy during exercise, but they also reduce training capacity because the body always burns some carbs during exercise and when those carbs are not adequately replenished, performance plummets.

The Zone Diet recommends that carbohydrates account for 40 percent of total calories. The typical endurance athlete gets 50 to 55 percent of his or her daily calories from carbohydrates. In 2002 researchers at Kingston University in England studied the effects of switching to the Zone Diet on high-intensity running endurance in a group of young men. Before the switch, the men were able to run for 37 minutes and

**TABLE 6.1 RECOMMENDED DAILY CARBOHYDRATE INTAKE BASED ON GOAL (RACING) WEIGHT**

| TRAINING VOLUME | CARBOHYDRATE INTAKE |
|---|---|
| ≤4 hours/week | 2–2.75 g/lb |
| 5–6 hours/week | 2.75–3.25 g/lb |
| 7–10 hours/week | 3.25–3.75 g/lb |
| 11–14 hours/week | 3.75–4 g/lb |
| 15–19 hours/week | 4–4.5 g/lb |
| 20–24 hours/week | 4.5–5 g/lb |
| ≥25 hours/week | 5–5.5 g/lb |

Note: Training intensity affects carbohydrate intake but not nearly to the degree that volume does, especially for endurance athletes. The recommendations above assume a typical training intensity distribution for endurance athletes. Few athletes train at intensities that are so far above or below the average as to render these guidelines inappropriate.

41 seconds on average at 80 percent of $VO_2$max. After a week on the Zone Diet that time had dropped all the way down to 34:06—a 9.5 percent decline in high-intensity running endurance.

It is worth pointing out that reducing carbohydrate intake has never been shown in any study to increase training capacity. Nor has increasing carbohydrate intake ever been shown to reduce training capacity. Increasing carbohydrate does not always increase training capacity, but it does under heavy training loads. The natural conclusion to draw from these facts is that endurance athletes should take pains to ensure that they are consuming enough carbohydrates to meet the demands imposed by their training load.

Most of us are familiar with carbohydrate intake guidelines in the form of recommendation percentages of total calories (such as the Zone Diet's 40 percent guideline). These recommendations are not very useful because they make carbohydrate intake dependent on total calorie intake, which is only marginally relevant to actual carbohydrate needs. Carbohydrate needs are actually dependent on body weight and activity level. Therefore, they should be expressed as absolute amounts (grams) rather than as percentages of daily calories.

Based on my review of the scientific literature, I suggest that you aim for a daily carbohydrate intake target that is based on your training workload as indicated by Table 6.1. Be sure to use your optimal racing weight instead of your current weight to make these calculations, as you're not trying to fuel your excess fat stores for optimal performance!

Many athletes with higher training loads are surprised by the large recommended carbohydrate intake values that result from Table 6.1 calculations. That's because the nutritional needs calculators that athletes may be familiar with do not account for how increasing training loads disproportionately increases carbohydrate needs versus fat and protein needs. Trust me, the numbers yielded by calculations based on Table 6.1 are valid. They are not absolute musts in all cases, however. If your carbohydrate intake is slightly lower than the amount recommended by this table, and your training and recovery are going very well, you may not notice any improvement after increasing your carb intake to the recommended level. Then again, you might.

One obvious implication of these recommendations is that not only should some endurance athletes eat more carbohydrates than others, but also any single endurance athlete's carbohydrate intake should vary as his or her training workload changes. If your training load increases, then your carbohydrate intake should rise, and if your training load drops, then your carbohydrate intake should also come down. The proportions of carbohydrates, fats, and proteins that nonathletes eat are as irrelevant to your body-weight management as an endurance athlete as they are to nonathletes' efforts to lose weight and prevent weight gain. All that matters in this regard is the total number of calories that are consumed daily.

### TABLE 6.2 HIGH-QUALITY, HIGH-CARBOHYDRATE FOODS

| FOOD | CARBOHYDRATE CONTENT |
|---|---|
| Bagel, whole wheat | 57 g |
| Banana | 25 g |
| Bread, whole wheat (2 slices) | 36 g |
| Breakfast cereal, whole grain (1 cup) | 45 g |
| Brown rice (1 cup) | 45 g |
| Lentils, cooked (1 cup) | 40 g |
| Oatmeal, old-fashioned (1 cup) | 25 g |
| Orange juice (1 cup) | 25 g |
| Potato, baked | 50 g |
| Spaghetti, whole wheat (1 cup) | 40 g |
| Tomato sauce (½ cup) | 22 g |
| Yogurt, lowfat with fruit (1 cup) | 50 g |

On the practical level of food selection, what does it take to meet your daily carbohydrate requirements? If your training load is moderate, it requires only that you include a few high-quality, high-carbohydrate foods in your daily nutrition regimen. If your training load is high, it may require such foods in every meal and snack throughout the day. Table 6.2 presents a selection of high-quality high-carbohydrate foods that you can rely on to meet your needs and the amount of carbs in each. Generally, the richest sources of carbohydrate are grains, dairy foods, legumes, and certain fruits (especially fruit juices).

# FAT AND PROTEIN

As I mentioned earlier, endurance athletes do not need as much fat or protein as carbohydrate and they are much less likely to fail to meet their fat and protein needs. Nevertheless, it's helpful to be acquainted with the minimal fat and protein requirements for optimal training performance.

## FAT REQUIREMENTS

The diet of the average American—which is also the diet of the average endurance athlete—is 30 to 35 percent fat. This is more than enough fat to support optimal training performance. The American College of Sports Medicine recommends that athletes aim to get a minimum of 20 percent of their calories from fat. However, a 2009 analysis of the diets of elite Kenyan runners revealed that on average they got only 13 percent of their calories from fat (Onywera, Kiplamai, and Pitsiladis 2004). Such real-world evidence suggests that a balanced diet of natural foods that supplies enough total energy will meet any person's fat needs, regardless of the specific numbers.

**DAILY DOSE: TAKE**

**2–3 g**
**OMEGA-3**
**FATS,**
or eat fish
3 times/week.

While few endurance athletes take in insufficient fat to meet their needs for that macronutrient, there is some evidence that athletes who try too hard to limit their fat intake fail to take in enough total energy to support their training, which may have negative consequences. A 2008 study of female runners found that those who ate the least fat had the highest injury rate (Gerlach et al. 2008).

One of the reasons that fat needs are low and easily met even in endurance athletes is that the body can readily convert excess carbohydrate to fat. But there are a few specific types of fats that the body cannot synthesize from other nutrients. These essential fats must be obtained directly from food. Some essential fats are classified as omega-6 fatty acids and others as omega-3 fatty acids. Omega-6 fatty acids are abundant in commonly eaten foods, but omega-3 fatty acids are not, and omega-3 fatty acid deficiency is widespread in our society. Omega-3 fatty acids play vital roles in the formation of healthy cell membranes, nerve cell function, and the formation of anti-inflammatory compounds in the body.

 A BALANCED DIET WILL MEET YOUR FAT NEEDS.

Preliminary research also suggests that omega-3 fatty acids may promote a lean body composition by enhancing the fat-burning effect of exercise (Hill et al. 2007). What's more, they may even boost aerobic exercise performance. A solid body of scientific research has shown that omega-3 fats increase the elasticity of the blood vessels, which improves circulation and lowers blood pressure. Omega-3 fats may boost cardiac efficiency during exercise through the same mechanism (Peoples et al. 2008).

The best food sources of omega-3 fats are certain types of fatty fish (wild salmon, herring, anchovies), flaxseeds, and flaxseed oil. Experts recommend consuming omega-3-rich fish at least twice a week to avoid deficiency. I recommend that everyone, regardless of how much fish he or she eats, take a daily essential fat supplement. The two most important omega-3 fats are DHA and EPA. A daily dosage of 2 to 3 grams of EPA and DHA (combined) is recommended.

As we've seen, some in the endurance sports community believe that athletes should not merely ensure that they meet their minimum fat requirement but should go out of their way to maintain a high-fat diet of around 40 percent of total calories. The rationale is that this teaches the muscles to rely on fat to fuel exercise, sparing precious glycogen stores and increasing endurance capacity.

Studies have found that increased fat intake does result in greater fat oxidation during exercise. Researchers from New Zealand compared the effects of a 14-day high-carbohydrate diet, a 14-day high-fat diet, and an 11.5-day high-fat diet followed by a 2.5-day carbo-loading diet on fat oxidation and performance in a 15-minute cycling test and a 100-km cycling test (Rowlands and Hopkins 2002). Performance in the 15-minute test was slightly better after the high-carb diet, but not to a statistically significant degree, while performance in the 100-km test was slightly better, but again not to a statistically significant degree, following the high-fat diet. Fat oxidation was significantly greater during the 100-km test following the high-fat diet.

By and large, studies of high-fat diets have found that they boost performance in only the longest tests of endurance while reducing performance in shorter, higher-intensity efforts. This was shown in a study from the University of Connecticut (Fleming et al. 2003). Twenty volunteers were divided into two groups and placed on either an endurance training program and a high-fat diet (consisting of 61 percent fat) or an endurance training program and a moderate-fat diet (consisting of 25 percent fat) for six weeks. They performed a $VO_2$max test and a 45-minute time trial before and after the study period. Members of the high-fat diet group exhibited a marked increase in fat burning during the 45-minute time trial, but their work output dropped by 18 percent relative to that of the moderate-fat group.

The greater problem with high-fat diets, as we have seen, is that they necessarily limit carbohydrate intake and thereby reduce training capacity. A diet cannot be both high fat and high carb. The benefits of a high-fat diet are small and the downside significant. The benefits of a high-carb diet are potentially large and the downside nonexistent.

So exactly how much fat should you eat? There's no need to put a number on it, except in the specific case of omega-3 fats. If you maintain a high-quality diet, consume enough total energy by eating according to your appetite, and consistently meet your carbohydrate needs, you will consume an appropriate amount of fat—neither too much nor too little.

## PROTEIN

According to the World Health Organization, the minimum protein requirement for good health is 10 percent of total calories. The average American gets 18 percent of daily calories from protein, and the typical endurance athlete does the same.

As with carbohydrate, it is somewhat misleading to express dietary protein requirements as a percentage of total calories. This is especially true for athletes because exercise increases carbohydrate needs more than it increases protein needs. According to the study I mentioned earlier, elite Kenyan runners get approximately 10 percent of their calories from protein. So it would appear that they are just barely meeting their minimum protein requirement. However, these athletes run 110 miles in a typical week. This training load greatly inflates their carbohydrate needs, which they meet by consuming a whopping 9.7 grams of carbs per kilogram of body weight daily. This massive carbohydrate intake diminishes the fractional contribution of protein to their total calories. But because the Kenyan runners' total energy intake is also very high, their absolute protein intake is also more than adequate.

**DAILY DIET:**
Athletes need about
**1.2 g**
OF PROTEIN/KG
BODY WEIGHT;

**1.3 g**
OF PROTEIN/KG
BODY WEIGHT
**for vegan athletes.**

There is a general consensus among researchers that athletes need to consume roughly 1.2 grams of protein per kilogram of body weight daily—compared to 0.8 g/kg for sedentary individuals—to meet basic health requirements and to adequately replace protein in the body that is broken down during and after workouts. The Kenyan runners whose diets were analyzed consumed an average of 1.3 grams of protein per kilogram of body weight.

It is not difficult to eat 1.2 grams of protein per kilogram of body weight in a day. A sizable majority of endurance athletes do. Although this minimum requirement is 50 percent greater than the requirement for nonathletes, the typical diet for nonathletes and endurance athletes alike provides between 1.3 and 1.4 grams of protein per kilogram of body weight.

The daily protein requirement for vegans is approximately 10 percent higher because the proteins in plant foods are less "bioavailable" than those in animal foods. So if you avoid all animal foods including dairy products, you'll want to aim for at least 1.3 grams of protein per kilogram of body weight daily. The irony of the higher protein requirement of vegans is that most plant foods contain far smaller amounts of protein than animal foods do. Nevertheless, with a little planning it is not at all difficult to get enough protein as a vegan athlete, and plenty of people do—most notably champion ultrarunner Scott Jurek, whose diet you can get a look at in Chapter 12.

It is best not to consume much more than your minimum requirement of protein because this will proportionally reduce your carbohydrate intake and possibly lower your training capacity. Researchers in New Zealand found that cycling time trial performance was significantly impaired by one week on a 30 percent protein diet (Macdermid and Stannard 2006).

There is a time for higher protein intakes in the life of an endurance athlete, and that's during the quick start period that precedes the beginning of a new race-focused training cycle. At this time fat loss becomes the top priority as performance recedes to second priority. Research has shown that high-protein diets increase fat loss and reduce muscle loss resulting from energy deficits. High-protein diets also attenuate the increase in hunger that typically accompanies an energy deficit. I'll say more about protein intake in quick start periods in Chapter 10.

# NO MAGIC RATIO

In the last years of the twentieth century and the first years of the twenty-first, our nation was gripped by a positive mania for weight-loss diets based on ratios of carbohydrate, fat, and protein. Every new diet that came along touted a new and supposedly better way of balancing energy sources—a certain magical macronutrient ratio—as the key to rapid and permanent weight loss. Nobody could agree on exactly what the perfect breakdown was, but everyone seemed certain that a perfect ratio of carbs, fat, and protein did exist.

The lack of agreement on the perfect ratio was the first clue that there was no perfect ratio. Research then made it abundantly clear that it is possible to manage weight effectively on a wide range of macronutrient ratios. Consequently, diets based on macronutrient ratios are not as trendy as they once were, but they have a legacy. Conscious eaters have been trained to be aware of the balance of energy sources in their diet.

I tried to make this point as clearly as I could in the first edition of this book, but I presented my guidelines for carbohydrate, fat, and protein intake in such a way that readers who wished to try calculating the exact percentages of their total calories should come from carbs, fat, and protein could. So I've changed the presentation of my guidelines to make such backdoor calculations of personal magical macronutrient ratios impossible.

To balance your energy sources appropriately to reach your optimal racing weight and maximize your performance, you do not need to know these percentages. You don't even need to know how many calories you need or consume. You will be assured of consuming the right amount of energy if you eat according to your appetite while maintaining high diet quality and practicing the appetite management techniques discussed in Chapter 5. You will be assured of meeting your carbohydrate requirements by following the guidelines in Table 6.1. This will maximize your training capacity and performance, which in turn will enhance all of the benefits of your training, including improvements in your body composition.

To meet your fat requirements you need only keep your diet quality up and eat fish at least twice a week and/or take a fish oil supplement. Finally, to get enough protein, count the number of protein grams you consume in a typical day and adjust your diet in the unlikely event that you're getting less than 1.2 g/kg of body weight if you're omnivorous and 1.3 g/kg if you're vegan.

That's all there is to it.

# SEVEN

STEP 4

# MONITORING YOURSELF

elf-monitoring plays an important role for endurance athletes seeking their racing weight. We've already looked at the cause side of the cause-effect equation of performance weight management. Monitoring your Diet Quality Score and your carbohydrate intake will ensure that your diet does not hold you back from attaining your racing weight. Remember, this desired effect—your optimal performance weight—is defined as your body weight and body composition when you're in peak racing form. Proper monitoring of the outcome of your diet and training therefore requires that you consistently track your body weight, body composition, and performance.

Competitive cyclists tend to be the most systematic of endurance athletes in their self-monitoring, and it frequently pays off. Consider Bradley Wiggins. Born in Belgium and raised in England, Wiggins got his start in the velodrome, where weight is not a handicap. His height of 6'3" and weight of 180 pounds were not impediments to his winning six Olympic medals in track cycling before becoming a full-time road racer.

Wiggins knew that in order to match his track success on the road circuit, he would have to lose weight. He created a plan with the aid of British Cycling coach Matt Parker that started with a goal weight of 158 pounds. This goal was based on calculations similar to those that I described in Chapter 2. Parker projected that 158 pounds was as light as Wiggins could get without losing any muscle mass or power and without lowering his body-fat level below the minimum amount needed for good health.

Then the tracking began. Wiggins weighed himself frequently and had his body composition measured regularly. But maintaining power and improving performance were no less important than losing fat, so Wiggins religiously tracked these variables as well. He repeated standard performance tests such as a 10-mile time trial to make sure he wasn't getting weaker as he got lighter. While he couldn't expect to become more powerful as a skinny roadie than he was as a beefy track specialist, he wanted to retain as much power as possible. The real goal was to improve his power-weight ratio, which would improve his climbing, so he also repeated a 30-minute climbing test.

The plan worked. Wiggins reached his weight goal at 4 percent body fat. He increased his average power to 475 watts in his 30-minute uphill time trial test. He was rewarded with a 4th-place finish in the 2009 Tour de France, wins at the Criterium du Dauphine in 2011 and 2012, and victories in the Tour de Romandie, Paris–Nice, and the Tour de France in 2012.

In your pursuit of racing weight, you'll want to track the same three variables that Bradley Wiggins does: weight, body-fat percentage, and performance. Let's start with the first two.

# TRACKING YOUR BODY WEIGHT

Some people believe that you shouldn't weigh yourself too often when you're trying to lose weight. They say that stepping on the scale causes unnecessary frustration because it's normal for a person's weight to sometimes hold steady or even creep upward a bit from one day to the next even when the general trend is downward. Opponents of frequent self-weighing also say that it encourages some people to adopt extreme and unhealthy measures to lose weight because they provide the only assurance that each day's bathroom scale reading will be smaller than the last one.

This perspective makes sense in theory, but the reality is very different. Research has shown that frequent self-weighing is one of the most common and effective weight-management strategies among men and women who have lost significant amounts of weight and kept it off. Frequency of self-weighing is a strong predictor of weight regain after initial weight loss. Dieters who weigh themselves more often regain less weight; those who weigh themselves less often regain more.

Studies have also demonstrated that the notion that frequent self-weighing causes mental anguish and encourages extremism is largely mythical. Daily weigh-ins are problematic for some individuals, but for most people they increase the chances of success without causing any psychological harm in the process.

There's no mystery to how self-weighing aids the prevention of weight regain. Without frequent weighing, it may take a month or more for a person who has gotten a bit slack with his diet and begun to regain weight to notice it through indicators such as waistband fit and the mirror test. A person who weighs himself every day, however, will catch the trend almost immediately and be able to take quick action to get his diet back up to standard.

There's really nothing to weighing yourself, but some people still manage to make a mess of it. I've known people who, whenever they are trying to lose weight, step on the scale two or three times a day and drive themselves crazy by making too much of any upward fluctuations, which are normal over the course of a day even when someone is successfully losing weight.

If, however, you still want to weigh yourself every day, you'll have research behind you to support this practice. In fact, a 2009 study involving men and women enrolled in a clinical weight-loss program found that, statistically, individual subjects lost an extra pound for every 11 times they weighed themselves, probably because of the heightened level of awareness that attends more frequent self-monitoring (Van Wormer et al. 2009). So if you wish to weigh yourself daily, go ahead; just be sure not to take daily fluctuations too seriously, and do weigh yourself at the same time each day and in the same circumstances for accurate comparisons. Don't weigh yourself first thing in the morning on the upstairs bathroom scale wearing pajamas one day and then weigh yourself after dinner on the downstairs bathroom scale in the nude the next day.

At a minimum, weigh yourself at least once every four weeks on the same day you perform your periodic fitness-test workouts (described later in this chapter). These are your "official weigh-ins" for use in determining your optimal performance weight.

Keep in mind that some scales are better than others. I suggest you invest in the best scale that's within your budget. One feature to look for is automatic zero calibration, which resets the scale to "true zero" weight after each use. You might also want a scale that gives readings to the ounce or tenth of a pound. Those little less-than-a-pound changes can be surprisingly motivating when you're pursuing your optimal performance weight. Finally, since you are also monitoring your body-fat percentage, it makes a lot of sense to purchase a scale that can give you feedback both on your weight and on your body composition.

## MEASURING YOUR BODY-FAT PERCENTAGE

Until fairly recently, there was no convenient, affordable, and accurate way to measure your own body-fat level. The best option available was the skinfold method, which entails pinching skinfolds between calipers and running the measurements through a complex mathematical formula. It was affordable enough but a hassle to do, and it was often inaccurate when performed without formal training. Hydrostatic (or underwater) weighing was considered the most accurate method, but it required bulky, expensive equipment that was not widely available.

Hydrostatic weighing has been replaced by DEXA scanning as the most accurate way to measure body-fat percentage, and in fact it is the only method that directly measures body-fat levels instead of estimating them based on measurements of other things. A DEXA scanner uses advanced imaging technology to "see" the body fat inside you (it is also used to measure bone mineral density). But getting a body-fat analysis from a DEXA scanner requires that you make an appointment with a doctor who has one, so it's no more convenient and affordable than hydrostatic weighing.

Thank goodness for body-fat scales! These use bioelectrical impedance technology for measurement and are now widely available at department stores, drugstores, sporting goods stores, and elsewhere. These devices are easy to use, affordable, and, while not as accurate as professional body-fat measurement methods such as DEXA scanning, accurate enough.

A 2007 study published in the journal *Clinical Nutrition* that compared measurements obtained from a Tanita body-fat scale and DEXA scanning reported a better than 96 percent level of agreement between the two methods (Thomson et al. 2007). Body-fat scales with this degree of accuracy are available for as little as $40.

Body-fat scales look just like regular bathroom scales. You step onto them and get a measurement. And they do in fact measure your body weight in addition to estimating your body-fat percentage. Body-fat scales work by sending an electrical signal into your body and measuring the degree of resistance (or impedance) encountered. Electrical signals pass through fat tissue more quickly than they do through muscle tissue, so the less resistance the body-fat scale registers, the higher your body-fat percentage must be.

To ensure accurate results, use your device in strict accordance with the instructions included with it. Different units have slightly different requirements. Here are some usage guidelines that apply to most body-fat scales:

- Always measure your body fat at the same time of day, preferably at least two hours after eating.
- Make sure you are well hydrated.
- Use the bathroom before stepping on the scale.
- Moisten a towel and step on it with bare feet before stepping on the scale (to enhance conductivity).
- Make sure the scale is on a flat, hard surface (such as bathroom tiles).

If you have good reason to believe that your body-fat percentage is already low (e.g., you have visible abdominal musculature), purchase a scale with an "athlete" mode. Scales without this feature are less accurate for lean individuals.

Popular brands of body-fat scales include Conair, Tanita (which also makes scales under the Weight Watchers, Ironman, and Jenny Craig brand names), Oregon Scientific, Phoenix, and Taylor. A company called Omron makes hand-held body-fat analyzers that use bioelectrical impedance as well, but these devices do not measure body weight. The difference between the higher-priced body-fat scales and the cheaper models is mainly in the number of features, not in their accuracy. You can find body-fat scales at department stores such as Wal-Mart, drugstores such as Walgreens, and sporting goods stores, including Sport Chalet.

Most of the fancier features on these devices have little or no value. For example, some devices purport to measure your hydration status.

This sounds like a useful tool for athletes, who are often dehydrated after workouts and must rehydrate fully to maximize performance in their next workout. But the accuracy of this feature is poor. What's more, the popular notion that endurance athletes commonly fail to properly rehydrate between workouts is false. An interesting study from the University of Glasgow, Scotland (Fudge et al. 2008), looked at the hydration status of elite Kenyan runners in heavy training over a five-day period. Despite becoming significantly dehydrated during their runs, and drinking little or nothing during or immediately after workouts, these runners were found to restore their bodies to normal hydration levels by the evening simply by drinking when thirsty throughout the day.

One fancy feature available in some body-fat scales that I do like is a basal metabolic rate calculator. This tool makes it easier to calculate the number of calories you burn each day, as you will do during your quick start periods (described in Chapter 10).

If you use a body-fat scale, you might as well measure your body-fat percentage as often as you measure your body weight, since you'll get both measurements from the same device. Note, however, that day-to-day fluctuations in body-fat percentage are perhaps even less meaningful than day-to-day changes in your body weight. The body-fat measurements that really matter are those that you calculate roughly once every four weeks, on the same day you do your fitness-test workouts, in the process of determining your optimal performance weight.

Again, body-fat scales are not the most accurate tools for measuring body-fat percentage. For this reason, it is best not to use them to compare your body composition to that of other people. But when your goal is simply to track changes in your own body-fat percentage, it's more important that your measurements be *consistent* (that is, your scale is measuring the same attribute to the same degree of accuracy on each occasion) than *accurate*, and body-fat scales do give consistent results when used properly. If the highest degree of accuracy is very important to you, there is a way to effectively increase the accuracy of your body-fat scale without taking on a lot of extra hassle or expense. Just make an appointment with a physician for a DEXA scan. Before you leave for that appointment, measure your body-fat percentage on your body-fat scale. Consider the difference between the two measurements the "margin of error" for your body-fat scale, and use that number to correct your scale's measurements going forward.

## KEEP YOUR DIET HONEST WITH A FOOD DIARY

**Weighing and body-fat measuring** are not the only forms of self-monitoring that are known to aid weight management. Keeping a food journal is another. Researchers at the Kaiser Permanente Health Research Center (Hollis et al. 2008) found that overweight individuals participating in an eight-month weight-loss program lost twice as much weight when they kept a daily food diary than when they logged their food intake irregularly or not at all.

You can keep your food diary anywhere—in a notebook, on a calendar, in a computer file—but I recommend keeping it in a place that goes everywhere you do, such as a smart phone. This way you can record the information when it's fresh in your memory and you'll be less likely to forget details or overlook entire meals!

Whereas self-weighing focuses on the effect side of the cause-effect equation of weight management, keeping a food journal sheds light on the cause side. Most people eat more food and have a lower-quality diet than they think they do. It's easy to fool yourself about your diet when you're not really paying attention. You eat one piece of fruit every other day and tell yourself you eat fruit often. You resist dessert once every ten days and tell yourself that you strictly limit your indulgence in sweets. When you keep a food diary, you're no longer able to fool yourself in these ways. You're forced to face the facts, and the facts give you an opportunity to make improvements that otherwise you probably would not make.

A food diary does not have to include calorie, macronutrient, or other nutrient counts to be effective. It's more likely to be effective if you keep it simple enough that it doesn't feel like a hassle. Your food diary should name everything you eat and drink in a day, broken down by occasion, in enough detail to allow for diet-quality scoring. Precise sizes are not necessary, but it's a good idea to include information about portions, especially when they are very small or very large. For example, if you eat a half a sandwich, it's better to write down "½ sandwich" instead of "sandwich."

For example, suppose your body-fat scale gives you a reading of 17.0 percent and the DEXA scanner gives you a reading of 18.8 percent (the DEXA scanner is almost certain to be higher, by the way). In all of your future body-fat scale measurements, add 1.8 percent to your reading to get your "true" body-fat percentage.

## MEASURING YOUR PERFORMANCE

Body weight and body-fat percentage have no meaning in isolation for endurance athletes. These variables have meaning only in relation to performance. Weighing 145 pounds is not better than weighing 155 pounds unless you perform better at the lighter weight. A body-fat percentage of 12 is better than a body-fat percentage of 13 only if you're faster at 12 percent.

> **WEIGHING 145 POUNDS IS NOT BETTER THAN WEIGHING 155 POUNDS UNLESS YOU PERFORM BETTER AT THE LIGHTER WEIGHT.**

Remember, optimal racing weight is defined as the body weight and body-fat percentage at which you perform best. Determining your racing weight requires that you track performance alongside your weight and body-fat percentage so that you know if the changes in your body are actually making you faster.

To determine your optimal performance weight, begin by creating a table that plots your body weight and body composition against your performance during a period of progressive training and carefully controlled diet in pursuit of a peak race performance. Once every four weeks, step on a body-fat scale and note your weight and body-fat percentage. On the same days you weigh in, perform a test workout that provides a good indicator of your race-specific fitness. For example, if you're a runner, go to the track and do a 10-km time trial at 95 percent effort.

Create a four-column table with the date in the farthest left column, your performance test time in the next column, your body weight in the next column, and your body-fat percentage in the far right column. After you've completed and recorded three or four testing days, you will begin to notice a clear pattern, as demonstrated in Table 7.1. It is likely that you will achieve your best performance at your lowest body weight and body-fat composition. And if you train and eat right, you will reach your highest performance level at the time of your scheduled peak race.

You're not done yet, however. Your weight at the time of your next peak race is not necessarily your optimal racing weight. If your current body-fat level is too high, you might not have enough time to reach your optimal performance weight by the date of your next peak race. And regardless of your starting weight, any one of a number of common training and dietary errors could prevent you from reaching your

**TABLE 7.1 TRACKING THE RACING WEIGHT MARKERS**

| DATE | PERFORMANCE TEST TIME (10K) | BODY WEIGHT (LBS.) | BODY FAT (%) |
|---|---|---|---|
| 3/9/13 | 43:02:00 | 141 | 22.1 |
| 4/6/13 | 42:29:00 | 137 | 21.0 |
| 5/4/13 | 41:58:00 | 136 | 20.7 |
| 6/1/13 | 42:30:00 | 134 | 20.2 |
| 6/29/13 | 40:43:00 | 130 | 19.7 |

optimal racing weight in time for your next peak race. If you're in this situation, you can't rely on your test workouts or race performances to tell you what your optimal performance weight is—yet. It may take you two or three full training cycles to arrive at the point where your performance is no longer limited by your weight. In this case your focus should be on consistently practicing the six-step Racing Weight plan, which will eliminate the dietary and training errors that are currently holding you back. In the meantime, keep tracking your weight, body-fat percentage, and performance so that you can watch and draw motivation from your progress along the way.

As you track your progress, measure *both* your body weight and your body-fat percentage because you can reach any given body weight at more than one body-fat percentage and in most endurance athletes body composition has an even stronger relationship to performance than body weight. If you track only body weight, you may wind up making the all-too-common mistake of approaching performance weight management with a simplistic "lighter is better" mentality and then trying to slim down in ways that cause you to lose muscle along with fat (most likely by undernourishing your body). Consequently, while you may eventually reach your optimal body weight through these means, you will do so at a greater-than-optimal body-fat percentage. Your performance at this body weight/body-fat percentage combination will not be as good as it is when you are at your optimal body weight *and* body composition (that is, your true optimal performance weight). Tracking your body-fat percentage along with your body weight can function as a check against making this mistake. Yes, you want to be light (unless, perhaps, you're a swimmer or rower), but you don't want to be light at all costs. You want to be light and lean.

Here's a concrete example of the process I've just outlined. A female runner completes five performance tests at four-week intervals spanning the duration of a full training cycle that begins with base training and culminates in a peak 10K race. Her performance test consists of a 10-km run on the track completed at a 95 percent effort level. She measures her body weight and body-fat percentage on the day of each performance test. Her results are seen in Table 7.1. Since her performance continues to improve as her body weight and body-fat percentage drop, she is able to conclude that she is moving toward her racing weight.

## PERFORMANCE TESTS

The following are suggested performance tests for the most popular endurance sports. Be sure to warm up properly for each of them.

**CROSS-COUNTRY SKIING.** Because snow conditions are ever changing and have a strong effect on cross-country skiing performance, it is seldom possible to do regular fitness tests outdoors on skis that provide a valid indication of changes in fitness. Therefore, I recommend that you use one of the following two alternatives instead.

*Option 1.* Ski as hard as you can for 20 minutes on a cross-country ski ergometer (an indoor ski machine with power-measuring capability). Note your average power output (watts).

*Option 2.* If you do not have regular access to a cross-country ski ergometer and you use cycling as a cross-training modality, perform the cycling test described below.

**CYCLING.** Ride 20 minutes at maximum effort on a flat, smooth road course or an indoor trainer. Note your distance covered, and use it to calculate your average speed or, if you use a power meter, note your average power. Whichever options you choose for your ride location and performance measurement variable, use them for every test for maximum validity of comparisons between tests.

**MOUNTAIN BIKING.** If your sport is mountain biking, you can use the cycling test described above or perform a 20-minute maximum effort on a stretch of trail that is easily accessed from your home. Be sure to ride the same stretch of trail every time you repeat the test.

**ROWING.** Perform a 5,000-meter time trial at maximum effort on a rowing ergometer. Note your time and calculate your average speed or note your average power output.

**RUNNING.** Run 10 kilometers at 95 percent of maximum effort on a running track or a smooth, flat road. Note your time, and calculate your average pace.

**SWIMMING.** Swim 5 × 100 meters on a 5:00 interval (with plenty of rest) in your main stroke discipline. Calculate your average time per 100 meters.

**SWIMMING (OPEN WATER).** If you want to use your performance test to prepare for open-water swimming, try one of the following options.

*Option 1.* Swim 1,000 meters at maximum effort in a pool. Note your time, and calculate your average pace per 100.

*Option 2.* Swim a marked open-water course that takes roughly 10 minutes to complete at maximum effort. Note your time. Be sure to swim in an area that is easily accessed from your home so that you can use it for all of your performance tests.

**TRIATHLON.** Each week perform one of the two cycling tests, the running test, or one of the two open-water swimming tests described above. Stagger the cycling and running tests so that you're never doing them in the same week. It's okay to do either the cycling and swimming tests or the running and swimming tests in the same week.

# MONITORING YOUR PROGRESS

In the corporate world, senior executives are fond of the expression "What gets measured gets managed." I like this expression, and I think it applies equally to health, fitness, and endurance performance. It expresses the idea that if you want to gain greater control over some aspect of your business (or your body), one of the best things you can do is to monitor it systematically using some kind of relevant measuring stick. The very effort to do so makes it a higher priority and helps you improve this aspect of your business or your body independently of other efforts.

You will find that estimating and tracking your progress toward your racing weight are similarly effective with respect to your objectives to become leaner and to maximize your race performance. Self-monitoring doesn't guarantee that you will always make progress, but even when your progress stalls, it will let you know that right away. You can then go back to the "cause" side of the cause-effect equation of performance management to see what you can do to start moving forward again, whether it's increasing your diet quality, filling holes in your training (see Chapter 9), or doing something else.

# EIGHT

STEP 5

# NUTRIENT TIMING

T. J. Tollakson could have been a bodybuilder, but he became a professional triathlete instead. After giving up soccer in college, Tollakson, in search of a new physical outlet, entered the popular Body-for-Life physique transformation contest. He lifted weights and ate a high-protein diet. His muscles grew so fast that he could almost see the transformation happening bit by bit. At the end of the 12-week contest, Tollakson was named a finalist. He weighed 200 pounds (at 5'10") when his "after" photos were taken.

Soon afterward Tollakson, who in addition to playing soccer had been a successful cross-country runner in high school, decided to do a triathlon. He knew he needed to lose weight to be competitive. Although his body-fat percentage was low, Tollakson understood that the excess muscle on his frame would slow him down just as much as an equal amount of excess body fat. He put himself on a 1,200-calories-a-day diet and lost 35 pounds in a matter of weeks.

A diet that supplies 1,200 calories a day is, of course, unsustainable for a competitive triathlete. After finding an ideal racing weight of 163 pounds, Tollakson went back to eating normally, always making sure he took in enough energy to support his training. But he had to be careful. While his exercise routine had changed, his genes had not. Tollakson still had a propensity to pack on muscle. The more he swam, the bigger he chest became; the more he rode his bike, the more his quadriceps inflated. Tollakson found himself sometimes gaining weight instead of losing it as he built up his training for races such as the Eagleman Ironman 70.3, which he won in 2007 and 2011, and Ironman Lake Placid, which he won in 2011.

Eating less was not an option for the strapping Iowan, and his diet quality was already very high. Tollakson ultimately found success in his performance weight management efforts not by changing how much or what he ate but rather by changing when he ate. He frontloaded his daily energy intake in accordance with the dictum "Eat breakfast like a king, lunch like a prince, and dinner like a pauper." He shifted around his macronutrients so that most of his carbohydrates were consumed before dinner and most of his protein was consumed in the evening. He became diligent in the practice of taking in recovery snacks immediately after workouts.

Tollakson often runs right after riding his bike, but he always squeezes some kind of snack into his transition between the two sessions. If he's home, he often eats peanut butter and jelly on toast. Otherwise, he gobbles an energy bar. As soon as he's *really* done training, Tollakson drinks a recovery smoothie while soaking in a cold bath. Heavy on dairy-based protein, the smoothie contains milk, Greek yogurt, whey protein powder, and frozen fruit.

Tollakson did not invent these practices. Many elite endurance athletes practice nutrient timing, as it is known, to maximize their training performance and recovery and manage their weight. It works as well for all who commit to it as it did for Tollakson. The beneficial effects of nutrient timing on body weight and body composition are also well documented in scientific literature. This is why timing nutrition is a part of the Racing Weight system.

## NUTRIENT TIMING FOR ENERGY PARTITIONING

The effects of nutrients on the body are usually ascribed to properties intrinsic to specific nutrients. Protein builds muscle, sugar causes an energy rush followed by an energy crash, and so forth. But this view is overly simplistic. The effects of nutrients on the body are actually determined as much by the context in which they are consumed as by their intrinsic properties. For example, protein is much more likely to become incorporated into muscle tissue in someone who regularly lifts weights than in someone who is inactive. In a person who lifts weights regularly, protein is much more likely to be incorporated into muscle tissue when consumed immediately after a workout than at any other time. And in a person who lifts weights regularly and has just completed a workout, protein is more likely to be incorporated into muscle tissue if it is consumed with carbohydrate than if it is consumed alone. (I'll explain why later in this chapter.)

As our example shows, there are three major contextual factors that influence the effects of specific nutrients on our bodies: the status of the body in which they are absorbed (weightlifter versus sedentary individual), the timing of the intake (after a workout versus at any other time), and other nutrients that are ingested at the same time (protein with carbohydrate versus protein alone). In this chapter we will focus on timing.

In simple terms, nutrient timing has a significant impact on *energy partitioning*. You may recall from the Introduction that energy partitioning refers to the ultimate fate of the calories your body absorbs from food. There are a few primary destinations for food calories:

- Fat may be stored in **ADIPOSE TISSUE**, making you fatter.
- Protein, carbohydrate, and fat may be stored within **MUSCLE CELLS** to power muscle work.
- Carbohydrate, fat, and, to a lesser extent, protein, may be used to supply **IMMEDIATE ENERGY NEEDS**.

Naturally, you become leaner by shifting the balance of energy partitioning away from fat storage and toward muscle storage and immediate use. If you time your nutrient intake well, you will store less fat in your fat cells, store more protein and carbohydrate in your muscle cells, and use more calories to supply immediate energy needs than you would if you ate precisely the same nutrients but timed their intake poorly.

Effective nutrient timing is a matter of pairing your intake of calories to your body's usage of calories throughout the day. Your body will tend to store body fat and lose muscle mass when you habitually eat more calories than your body needs to meet its energy demands for the next few hours and also—counterintuitively—when you take in *fewer* calories than you need to meet short-term energy requirements. On the one hand, when you take in too much, your body stores most of the excess as fat in adipose tissue. On the other hand, when you habitually consume too little at certain times of the day, your metabolism will slow so that more of the calories you consume at other times are stored as body fat, and your body will break down muscle tissue to make up for the deficit of food energy.

This negative effect of short-term food-energy deficits on body composition was shown in a study involving elite female gymnasts and distance runners, which found a strong inverse relationship between the number and size of energy deficits throughout the day (that is, periods when the body's calorie needs exceeded the calorie supply from foods) and body-fat percentage (Deutz et al. 2000). In other words, the athletes who did the best job of matching their calorie intake with their calorie needs throughout the day were leaner than those who tended to fall behind.

Your body's energy requirements are not consistent throughout the day. They are much greater at some times than at others. To practice nutrient timing effectively, you must maintain an eating schedule that anticipates and responds to these fluctuations in energy needs. Here are seven rules of nutrient timing that you can use to match your calorie intake with your body's calorie needs throughout the day.

**RULE 1**  **EAT EARLY.** Numerous studies have shown that regular breakfast eaters tend to be leaner than regular breakfast skippers, but the reasons may surprise you. You have probably heard and read a thousand times that you should eat a good breakfast because doing so will rev up your metabolism so that you burn more calories throughout the day. In fact, however, there is very little scientific evidence for such an effect. A 2008 review published in the *Journal of International Medical Research* (Giovannini et al. 2008) did not include increased metabolism on a list of three possible mechanisms by which eating breakfast may promote a healthy body weight. The researchers did, however, identify three mechanisms other than metabolic increase that may explain why starting the day with breakfast is a good idea.

Overall reduced appetite and reduced eating throughout the day (really just two facets of a single mechanism) are both outcomes of eating breakfast. Less overall appetite is experienced throughout the day when a person eats early in the day compared to waiting longer to eat the first

## EATING FOR EARLY WORKOUTS

**If you plan to work out** more or less immediately after waking, your preworkout nutrition should consist of a small dose of easily absorbed carbs and little else. Eight ounces of sports drink, an energy gel, or a banana will do the trick. If you have an hour or so to get ready, something more substantial—but still high in carbs and low in protein and fat—will give you an even greater lift. Consider a 12- to 16-ounce fruit smoothie, 6 to 8 ounces of low-fat yogurt, or a small bowl of oatmeal.

meal. Men and women who eat little or not at all in the morning wind up very hungry in the afternoon and evening, and as a result they overeat, more than making up for the "fasting" they did earlier in the day. A study from the University of Texas–El Paso (De Castro 2007) found that the fewer calories subjects ate early in the day, the more total calories they ate during the day as a whole.

Improved diet quality is another potential mechanism connecting breakfast with leaner body composition. Research has shown that regular breakfast eaters typically eat more high-quality foods and fewer low-quality foods than regular breakfast skippers. This is harder to explain. More than likely, regular breakfast eaters are more conscientious eaters generally, and both their breakfast eating habit and their selection of quality foods are manifestations of their conscientiousness. In my own experience I have found that eating breakfast promotes a higher-quality diet by giving me another opportunity to work toward eating my daily quota of high-quality foods (my typical breakfast is whole-grain cereal with fresh berries and organic whole milk, orange juice, and black unsweetened coffee) and by keeping my appetite under control throughout the morning. That way, I am less likely to eat low-quality foods later, as the hungrier I am, the harder it is for me to resist the temptation of junk food.

Another benefit of eating early that is specific to endurance athletes who train in the morning is that it boosts performance and thereby enhances the training effects of the workout, including its overall fat-burning effect. When you wake up in the morning, your liver is approximately 50 percent glycogen depleted owing to having powered your nervous system as you slept. Endurance capacity is related to liver glycogen content, so your endurance capacity is reduced after the overnight fast. This is no big deal if you are doing a light workout; you won't be limited even if you eat or drink nothing before starting it. But if your morning workout will be taxing, you will perform at a higher level by consuming some calories before starting.

**RULE 2** **EAT CARBS EARLY AND PROTEIN LATE.** In their 2011 book, *Hardwired for Fitness*, Robert Portman, a biochemist who has developed a number of ergogenic products for endurance athletes, and John Ivy, a respected exercise physiologist at the University of Texas, argued that the macronutrient needs of athletes are not fixed throughout the day. While the overall diet should be relatively high in carbohydrate, the body's need for carbohydrate is proportionally even greater in the early part of the day. Protein, on the other hand, is most needed late in the day. Eating in accordance with these fluctuating needs will promote favorable nutrient partitioning and a leaner body composition.

Carbohydrate needs are elevated in the morning because, as already described, liver glycogen stores have been depleted during the night. People tend to be most active in the morning as well, and carbohydrate is the nutrient best able to supply immediate energy requirements. Athletes who work out in the morning need an early dose of carbs especially. Because the body is hormonally "primed" to convert dietary carbs to energy in the early part of the day, it does so more efficiently than it does later in the day. Carbs consumed at night are more likely to be converted to fat and stored.

Another thing to consider is that cortisol levels are high in the morning, and exercise brings them even higher. Cortisol is a "catabolic" hormone that breaks down fats, carbs, and protein for energy. Without cortisol you couldn't swim, bike, or run very fast. But when cortisol levels get too high, a lot of muscle protein is broken down, compromising recovery. Consuming carbs before and during morning workouts lowers cortisol levels and helps recovery.

There's nothing intrinsically wrong with eating high-protein foods for breakfast. It's just that you can only eat so much and carbs are more important at this time. Also, the synthesis of proteins inside the body from amino acids derived from protein in food requires energy—energy that is best reserved for your daily activities and training in the first part of the day.

Many traditional breakfast foods—including cold cereal, oatmeal, bagels, and fruit smoothies—are high in carbs. These are excellent choices for your breakfasts as an endurance athlete. Dinner is another story. In the evening the body switches from energy supply mode to tissue rebuilding mode. Protein is the raw material for tissue rebuilding. Nutrient timing is all about supplying your body with what it needs when it needs it. Concentrating your protein intake in the latter part of the day will maximize muscle regeneration in the evening and through the night. Over time such favorable energy partitioning will make you leaner than if you ate more protein for breakfast and lunch and more carbs at dinner.

> CONCENTRATING PROTEIN INTAKE LATER IN THE DAY WILL MAXIMIZE MUSCLE REGENERATION IN THE EVENING AND THROUGH THE NIGHT.

Again, from day to day your diet should have a consistent balance of macronutrients that favors carbohydrate, but ideally this will not be the macronutrient balance of every meal. For example, let's suppose that your normal diet is 65 percent carbohydrate and 15 percent protein. In this case your breakfast should be closer to 80 percent carbs and 10 percent protein, your lunch 65 percent carbs and 15 percent protein, and your dinner 50 percent carbs and 25 percent protein. The exact numbers don't matter. What's important is that you make some effort to frontload your daily carbohydrate consumption and backload your protein intake while maintaining the right overall balance of macronutrients from day to day.

**RULE 3** **EAT ON A CONSISTENT SCHEDULE.** How many times a day should you eat? Three times? Four times? More? There is no single optimal meal frequency for everyone. While three meals a day seems to be a universal minimum requirement for controlling appetite and maintaining energy levels, whether it is necessary to eat one or more snacks in addition to breakfast, lunch, and dinner is an individual matter. Even though a "grazing" approach to diet is recommended by many diet authorities, the results of research on its effects are equivocal, and in the real world many successful endurance athletes, including Olympic and World Championships bronze medalist Shalane Flanagan, seldom snack between meals.

There is a popular belief that eating frequently increases metabolism and thereby promotes weight loss, but research does not support such a mechanism. A 2008 study by Dutch researchers compared the outcomes of normal-weight women who spent 36 hours in a metabolic chamber under two different conditions (Smeets and Westerterp-Plantenga 2008). In one session they consumed two meals per 24-hour period, and in the other they consumed three meals. Measurements taken in the two sessions revealed no differences in either resting metabolic rate or the amount of energy subjects expended through voluntary activity.

This study was limited by its short duration and the small difference in the number of meals eaten. It did not rule out the possibility that metabolic rate increases as a long-term adaptation to greater eating frequency or that those who habitually eat 6 times a day have a higher resting metabolic rate than those who eat just 2.7 times per day, as the average person does. But other studies have addressed the limitations of the Dutch study. For example, an interesting study by undergraduate researchers at the University of Wisconsin–La Crosse (Goodman-Larson, Johnson, and Shevlin 2003) compared the resting metabolic rate and eating frequency of 22 women on their habitual diets. Statistical analysis revealed no correlation between the two variables.

RESEARCH HAS SHOWN THAT EATING ON THE SAME SCHEDULE EVERY DAY IS MORE IMPORTANT THAN EATING MORE FREQUENTLY THROUGHOUT THE DAY.

Grazing is also recommended on the grounds that it reduces appetite and total calorie intake over the course of a day. This idea appears to be a myth as well. In 2011 researchers at the University of Missouri analyzed past studies addressing the effects of meal frequency on appetite and food intake (Leidy and Campbell 2011). They found that reducing meal frequency below the standard three meals a day caused a significant increase in appetite and a tendency to overeat at the next meal. However, increasing meal frequency above the standard three meals a day had minimal effects on appetite control. In other words, increasing your meal frequency is likely to strengthen your appetite control only if you currently eat just once or twice a day.

What seems to be more important than eating a certain number of times every day is eating on the same schedule every day. In other words, once you've found a daily eating schedule that works for you, whether it entails three meals a day or three meals and three snacks, stick with it. Research has demonstrated a few advantages of a consistent eating schedule. A 2004 study by British scientists found that two weeks on a diet characterized by irregular meal frequency increased blood lipid levels and reduced insulin sensitivity in lean, healthy women (Farschi, Taylor, and Macdonald 2004b). A companion study involving the same subjects found that regular meal frequency increased the thermic effect of food, or the spike in metabolism that followed eating, compared to irregular meal frequency (Farschi, Taylor, and Macdonald 2004a). Together these effects indicate that an erratic eating schedule likely creates energy partitioning that favors fat storage while a consistent eating schedule creates partitioning that favors immediate energy use and muscle maintenance.

Determining your optimal eating schedule requires a little experimentation. It does not, however, require invasive measurements of insulin sensitivity and metabolic rate. You can simply go by feel. The factors to consider are appetite, energy level, and the effect of eating on your workouts. If you find that you cannot keep hunger at bay on three meals a day, you may need to snack. Nibbling between meals may also be necessary if your energy level plummets between breakfast and lunch or between lunch and dinner. If you perform poorly in late-morning workouts undertaken a few hours after breakfast or in late-afternoon workouts undertaken a few hours after lunch, snacking may correct the problem. If, however, you tend to experience gastrointestinal discomfort when you exercise too soon after eating, it may be best to avoid snacking.

While your eating schedule should be consistent from day to day, be open to adjusting your habitual meal frequency in response to changes in your training and appetite. During periods of moderate training I seldom get hungry between meals and snack once a day at most. At the height of training for marathons or triathlons, however, I'm hungry all the time and routinely eat three snacks a day in addition to three meals. What I don't do is arbitrarily bounce around between the extremes of three and six meals from one day to the next.

**RULE 4** **EAT BEFORE EXERCISE.** Eating before exercise is a nutrient timing method that will help you reach and maintain your racing weight in two ways. First, it will enhance your workout performance and thereby enhance the results you get from workouts, including that of fat burning. Second, it will directly affect your body composition by increasing the number of food calories you burn and decreasing the number of calories you store.

It is not a good idea to eat a full meal immediately before working out, of course. The jostling that a full stomach undergoes during vigorous exercise may cause gastrointestinal distress. And even if it doesn't, your workout performance is likely to be compromised by the shunting of blood flow to the gut, and away from the extremities, which normally occurs after a meal. The ideal time for a pre-exercise meal to maximize workout performance is two to four hours out. Four hours allows enough time for a large meal to clear the stomach but not so much that liver glycogen and blood sugar levels begin to drop. Two hours allows enough time for a medium-sized meal to clear the stomach.

Carbohydrate is the most important nutrient to consume in a pre-exercise meal. To maximize performance, aim to consume at least 100 grams of carbohydrate within the four hours preceding a hard workout. It does not matter whether these carbs come from high-glycemic (i.e., rapidly absorbed) food sources or low-glycemic (i.e., slowly absorbed) food sources. Studies indicate that there is no difference in their effects on subsequent exercise performance. That said, most or all of your carbs should come from high-quality foods for the simple reason that eating high-quality foods generally will help you get lean and stay lean.

WHEN THE MUSCLES BURN MORE CARBOHYDRATE DURING A WORKOUT, THEY TEND TO BURN MORE FAT AFTER THE WORKOUT.

Within these parameters, the precise timing and composition of the pre-exercise meal that works best are an individual matter. Most athletes naturally find a routine that suits them. To find the routine that works best for you, pay attention to how your gastrointestinal system feels and to your energy level and performance after meals of different sizes and compositions eaten at different times before exercise and heed your body's messages.

In most circumstances the timing and composition of your prework-out meals should be optimized for performance. Nonathletes are some-times coached to work out within an hour after eating for the sake of other benefits, including increased calorie burning (Davis et al. 1989), reduced fat storage (Aoi et al. 2012), and reduced appetite (Martins et al. 2007). While there is research to support these benefits, they are not relevant to endurance athletes. As an endurance athlete you will gain greater improvements in body composition by focusing on eating for performance.

The exception to this rule occurs within quick starts, when fat loss becomes a higher priority than performance. During quick starts I rec-ommend weekly fat-burning workouts that are performed early in the day on an empty stomach. While you won't perform as well in these workouts, you will burn more fat.

**RULE 5** **EAT DURING EXERCISE.** It is seldom necessary or practical to eat solid food during exercise, but it is beneficial to drink and consume semisolids such as energy gels. Scores of studies have demonstrated that performance in harder workouts and races is enhanced by the consump-tion of water, carbohydrate, and, to a lesser extent, protein or amino acids. Consuming these nutrients regularly in your harder workouts will help you become leaner by enhancing the training effects that you derive from them, including that of fat burning.

Some endurance athletes limit their consumption of calories during workouts for fear that using a sports drink or carbohydrate gel will cancel out the calorie-burning effect of training and impede their efforts to shed excess body fat. But in fact calories—specifically carbohydrates—con-sumed during workouts are canceled out by reduced calorie intake after workouts. A study conducted at Colorado State University found that when subjects consumed no carbohydrate during a workout, they ate 777 calories at their next meal (Melby et al. 2002). But when they took in 45 grams of carbs during a workout, they ate only 683 calories in their next meal. What's more, the subjects consumed fewer total calories—includ-ing workout carbs—during the day in which they exercised with carbs than they did during the day when they exercised without carbs.

Consuming carbohydrate during exercise increases the muscles' reli-ance on carbs as fuel and decreases their reliance on fat. Therefore less fat

## HOW TO EAT AROUND A WORKOUT

| 2-4 HRS. PRIOR | WORKOUT | WITHIN 2 HRS. |
|---|---|---|
| **CARBS** | **HYDRATION + CARBS** | **HYDRATION, CARBS + PROTEIN** |
| Meal high in carbohydrates | For workouts over 2 hours or high-intensity workouts, consume carbohydrates (e.g., sports drink, energy gels + water) | Meal replenishing both carbohydrates and protein |
| **+100** g CARBS | **30–60** g CARBS/hr. | **1.2** g CARBS/kg body weight + **1** g PROTEIN/ 4 g carbs |

is burned during a workout in which a sports drink or gel product is used than in an identical workout in which the athlete drinks only water or goes thirsty. This is another reason some endurance athletes limit their use of sports drinks and carbohydrate gels in training. However, when the muscles burn more carbohydrate during a workout, they tend to burn more fat after the workout. In the Colorado State study the lesser amount of fat burning that occurred during the workout done with carbohydrate intake was almost completely compensated for by greater fat burning after the workout compared to the workout done without carb intake.

At the end of the day what matters is not what kind of calories you burned during your workout but how many calories you burned. You will tend to burn more calories in harder workouts when you consume carbs because it will elevate your performance. Like the matter of general carbohydrate intake that we discussed in Chapter 4, carb intake during workouts is another matter where you can trust that doing what's best for your performance will also yield the best results for your body composition.

It is not necessary to take in carbohydrate in every workout. Only longer and faster workouts challenge the body enough for carb intake to make a difference in performance. As a general rule, any workout lasting longer than two hours and any high-intensity workout lasting longer than one hour will be aided by carb intake. Aim to take in at least 30 grams of carbs per hour and up to 60 grams per hour.

It is advisable to drink according to thirst and stomach comfort to minimize dehydration and its effects on performance in challenging workouts as well. A sports drink addresses both fluid and carbohydrate needs, but drinking according to thirst and comfort may not provide enough carbohydrate to maximize performance, especially during running, an activity in which tolerable drinking rates are lower. In such cases you'll want to supplement with carbohydrate gels. You may also choose to rely on carbohydrate gels entirely to meet your carbohydrate needs. In this scenario you'll want to hydrate with plain water or an electrolyte-fortified water.

Research has shown that there are benefits associated with consuming a small amount of protein along with carbohydrate during challenging workouts. Protein appears to delay fatigue by mechanisms that are partly independent of those by which carbohydrate works. Consequently, sports drinks and gels containing carbs and protein are more effective calorie for calorie than those that exclude protein. A study conducted at the University of Texas and published in 2010 found that a carbohydrate-protein sports drink (Accelerade Hydro) with 55 percent fewer calories per serving than Gatorade improved endurance performance as much as Gatorade (Martinez-Lagunas et al. 2010). The addition of protein to sports drinks and carbohydrate gels is also proven to reduce muscle damage during challenging workouts and thereby improve performance in a subsequent workout compared to conventional drinks and gels.

**RULE 6**  **EAT AFTER EXERCISE.** Eating soon after exercise is completed also promotes leanness both directly and indirectly. It promotes leanness directly by shifting energy partitioning toward muscle protein and glycogen synthesis and away from body-fat storage. It does so indirectly by accelerating muscle recovery so that an athlete can perform at a higher level in the next workout and derive a stronger training effect from it. How soon is soon? Research has identified a two-hour postexercise nutritional recovery window. What this means is that recovery proceeds significantly faster if the right nutrients are consumed less than two hours after exercise than if precisely the same nutrients are consumed more than two hours after exercise. But it is generally agreed that even within this window, the sooner you eat or drink, the better.

The most important nutrients to consume after exercise are carbohydrate for replenishing muscle and liver glycogen stores, protein for repairing and remodeling muscles, and water for rehydrating. For the best results, aim to consume at least 1.2 grams of carbohydrate per kilogram of body weight in the first several hours after exercise (beginning within the first hour), along with roughly 1 gram of protein per 4 grams of carbohydrate and enough water (or other fluid) so that your urine is pale yellow or clear within a few hours after the workout is completed. Again, timing is important. In a study conducted by John Berardi and colleagues,

**TABLE 8.1 TIMING YOUR DAILY NUTRITION**

| NUTRITION TIMING | MORNING | | | |
|---|---|---|---|---|
| **MORNING** WORKOUT | **Pre-workout snack** Small amount of an easily absorbed HIGH-CARB FOOD OR DRINK | **WORKOUT** SPORTS DRINK according to thirst | **BREAKFAST** Postworkout recovery High CARB Moderate PROTEIN Low FAT | **Midmorning snack** *(optional)* |
| **MIDDAY** WORKOUT | **BREAKFAST** Balance of high-quality foods; emphasis on CARBS | | | **Pre-workout snack** High CARB Moderate PROTEIN Low FAT |
| **AFTERNOON** WORKOUT | **BREAKFAST** Balance of high-quality foods; emphasis on CARBS | | | **Midmorning snack** *(optional)* |
| **TWO** WORKOUTS DAILY | **Pre-workout snack** Small amount of an easily absorbed HIGH-CARB FOOD OR DRINK | **WORKOUT** SPORTS DRINK according to thirst | **BREAKFAST** Postworkout recovery High CARB Moderate PROTEIN Low FAT | **Pre-workout snack** *(optional)* |

*Note:* Meals that are part of postworkout recovery are emphasized to reflect the body's demand for more calories.

cyclists were found to have synthesized 55 percent more muscle glycogen six hours postexercise when they consumed a carbohydrate-protein supplement immediately, one hour, and two hours after exercise and then ate a small meal four hours after exercise, than when they consumed the same total number and types of calories in a larger meal consumed four hours after exercise (Berardi et al. 2006).

In this particular study, the different nutritional protocols and their disparate effects on muscle glycogen replenishment had no effect on performance in a subsequent one-hour time trial, but in other, similar studies better postexercise nutrient timing and muscle glycogen replenishment boosted subsequent exercise performance (Williams et al.

| MIDDAY | | AFTERNOON | | EVENING | |
|---|---|---|---|---|---|
| **LUNCH**<br>Balance of high-quality foods | | **Midafternoon snack**<br>*(optional)* | | **DINNER**<br>Balance of high-quality foods; emphasis on PROTEIN | **Evening snack**<br>*(optional)* |
| **WORKOUT**<br>SPORTS DRINK according to thirst | **LUNCH**<br>**Postworkout recovery**<br>High CARB<br>Moderate PROTEIN<br>Low FAT | **Midafternoon snack**<br>*(optional)* | | **DINNER**<br>Balance of high-quality foods; emphasis on PROTEIN | **Evening snack**<br>*(optional)* |
| **LUNCH**<br>Balance of high-quality foods | | **Pre-workout snack**<br>High CARB<br>Moderate PROTEIN<br>Low FAT | **WORKOUT**<br>SPORTS DRINK according to thirst | **DINNER**<br>**Postworkout recovery**<br>High CARB<br>Moderate PROTEIN<br>Low FAT | |
| **LUNCH**<br>Balance of high-quality foods | | **Pre-workout snack**<br>High CARB<br>Moderate PROTEIN<br>Low FAT | **WORKOUT**<br>SPORTS DRINK according to thirst | **DINNER**<br>**Postworkout recovery**<br>High CARB<br>Moderate PROTEIN<br>Low FAT | |

2003). Habitually consuming carbs, protein, and fluid soon after completing workouts will generally lift your performance and accelerate your fitness gains, which, again, occur primarily through the recovery process.

Proper postexercise nutrition also promotes fat burning. A meal eaten after exercise has a very different effect on the body than a meal eaten at any other time. No matter when you eat, your metabolism increases, because your body has to burn calories to digest and absorb food. But this "thermic effect of food" is greater when the food is consumed after exercise. More important, however, is the type of calories your body burns. When a meal is not preceded by exercise, carbohydrate burning increases most. But when a meal does follow exercise, fat burning increases while carbohydrate is spared so that it can be delivered to the muscles to replenish depleted glycogen stores. Thus, an athlete who routinely eats within an hour after working out will burn a little more fat and store a little more glycogen each day, and eventually she or he will wind up a little leaner than an athlete who routinely waits two hours after working out to chow down.

Not only is more fat burned, but also more muscle is built or preserved when a meal is consumed soon after exercise, as long as that meal includes both carbohydrate and protein. Several studies have shown that individuals engaged in strength training programs gain significantly more muscle when they consume carbohydrate and protein immediately after exercise instead of waiting to eat. While most endurance athletes have no interest in adding weight of any kind to their bodies, every endurance athlete benefits from maximizing his or her muscle-to-fat ratio at any given weight. Studies showing that endurance athletes build more new muscle proteins when they consume carbohydrate and protein immediately after exercise offer reason to believe that this nutrient timing practice helps endurance athletes maximize their muscle-to-fat ratio.

RULE 7 **MINIMIZE EATING AFTER DARK.** Our bodies are clocks. Recent advances in understanding circadian rhythm, or the 24-hour cycle of sleep and wakefulness and related processes, have revealed that the functioning of our bodies is affected far more extensively by circadian rhythm than was previously known. We now know that 1 out every 10 genes in human DNA operates in a 24-hour cycle. Many of these genes affect metabolism.

Our circadian hardwiring causes the same foods to be metabolized in different ways depending on when they are eaten. If first thing in the morning is the best time to eat, late at night may be the worst. Research suggests that exposure to artificial light at night disrupts natural circadian rhythms in ways that influence the timing of food intake, alter metabolism, and promote weight gain. Mice housed in a constantly lit environment eat more at night and are significantly fatter than mice housed in an environment with a natural light/dark cycle, despite eating the same total number of calories and burning the same number of calories through activity.

You're not a mouse, of course, and it is difficult to perform this kind of controlled experiment in humans to determine whether what's true for mice in this case it true for us. But there is reason to believe it is, because nightshift workers are known to be fatter than dayshift workers. So try to restrict your eating after sundown.

The overall body of research on the effects of nighttime eating on body weight and body composition in humans indicates that a habit of snacking in the evening does not automatically sabotage efforts to get leaner. The evidence that eating breakfast is good for weight management is much stronger than the evidence that nighttime eating is bad.

It is noteworthy, however, that many successful endurance athletes strictly limit their snacking after dark in the interest of attaining their racing weight. Triathlete Peter Reid, in addition to keeping an empty kitchen, as we saw in Chapter 5, once confessed that during the run-up to a big race he often went to bed so hungry he had a headache. I don't think that's quite necessary for most of us. T. J. Tollakson has said he tries to go to bed "mildly hungry." That sounds better.

Of course, if you need a snack at night to avoid going to bed so hungry that you can't sleep, go for it. At this time a high-protein snack is best; remember, your body is in rebuilding mode at the end of the day, and protein supports this metabolic objective. A 2012 study by Dutch researchers reported that a high-protein snack consumed at bedtime after strenuous exercise increased overnight muscle protein synthesis (Res et al. 2012). It's all about giving your body what it needs when it needs it.

# NINE

STEP 6

# TRAINING FOR RACING WEIGHT

Georgia Gould did not worry much about her weight during her first two seasons as a professional mountain bike racer in 2004 and 2005. When she lost a few pounds before the start of her third season, which was her first as a member of the LUNA team, it wasn't because she tried to. The weight loss was simply an effect of stepped-up training.

After winning her first national championship later that year, however, Gould couldn't help but associate her improved performance (she won a number of other races in 2006 as well) with her drop in weight. Gould started to give her weight and her food intake more attention than she had in the past. Even a single pound of gain concerned her, and while she knew better than to undereat, she tried hard to limit her intake to what she considered "barely enough."

Eventually, Gould realized that her constant worrying about calories, pounds, and ounces was draining a lot of the enjoyment out of her eating. An avid cook, she decided that if joyless eating was what it took to stay lean and to win, she would rather enjoy eating and lose. So she continued to eat very healthily but went back to eating enough to feel completely satisfied. And she stayed lean and kept on winning.

Subsequent experience taught Gould that it was really the training that had made her leaner and improved her racing. A healthy diet was something that was always there for her. But when her training slipped for any reason, she tended to put on a bit of fat, whereas when she got into a good groove with her training, the fat disappeared.

Gould's favorite type of workout is a long tempo ride—three or four hours with lots of sustained efforts close to lactate threshold intensity. When she gets a few of these rides in her legs at the beginning of a new season or during a break between races, she can feel her fitness improving almost from one day to the next. Long tempo rides also move her more quickly toward her racing weight than any other type of training.

This is no coincidence. The most effective training for improved endurance performance is also the most effective training for a lean body composition. Endurance athletes are the leanest athletes. Sure, endurance sports select for naturally leaner individuals, but it's the training above all that makes cyclists, swimmers, runners, and triathletes leaner than ball players. In a typical workout an endurance athlete raises his or her metabolic rate 8- to 16-fold and keeps it there for a long time. There's no more efficient way to burn calories.

That is why many nonathletes exercise more or less like endurance athletes when their goal is to lose weight. As an endurance athlete you should not train specifically for weight loss, however. In other words, you don't want to change your training for the sake of shedding more fat without regard for how the changes will affect your performance. You should train for performance and trust that your body will move toward racing weight as your fitness moves toward peak level. The one exception to this rule is the quick start period that falls outside of race-focused training, when fat loss briefly supplants performance as your top priority and you modify your diet and training accordingly. Within a race-focused training cycle, however, every decision you make about how much you train, how intensely, and so forth should be made exclusively for the sake of better performance. If you do, you will discover, as Georgia Gould did, that what's best for performance is best for body composition.

WORKOUTS CAN **BOOST METABOLISM** TO AS MUCH AS *16 TIMES* its normal rate.

# WHAT WORKS

The modern sports of bicycle racing, running, and swimming have existed since the late nineteenth century. Triathlon started in the 1970s, but since it comprises swimming, cycling, and running, it's not really as new as other sports of the same vintage. The training methods of today's top endurance athletes are very different from those of the early competitors in the various disciplines. These methods have evolved as innovative techniques have yielded better results and then spread throughout the sport to become universal practices.

Innovation in training methods has slowed considerably since the 1960s. In each sport athletes have figured out what works and are now focused on just doing it. The occasional good idea or new trend comes along, but these affect the margins only. One hundred twenty years ago most distance runners trained by walking. Then they figured out that running worked better. It's been a while since a shakeup of that magnitude appeared.

Interestingly, despite the obvious differences among the individual endurance sports, the best athletes in all endurance sports train in fundamentally the same way. We can see this when we look at training mathematically. A number of years ago Stephen McGregor, an exercise scientist at Eastern Michigan University, co-developed a set of mathematical tools to quantify the physiological stress imposed by swimming, cycling, and running workouts. One of these tools, called Chronic Training Load (CTL), is a rolling average of an athlete's training stress, including duration and intensity of workouts, over the previous several weeks.

Thousands of endurance athletes around the world, including many world-class athletes, track their CTL with McGregor's software. A while back McGregor began to notice that peak CTL scores tended to fall in the same range—between 120 and 140—for elite cyclists, runners, and triathletes, and he was able to estimate that the pattern held for swimmers too. This pattern suggests that there is a maximum amount of aerobic training stress that the human body can tolerate and that endurance athletes perform best when they hug that threshold without exceeding it. Athletes in different disciplines get there in slightly different ways, and most don't do it consciously, but they all get there because it works.

It takes a very high volume of training to reach a CTL of 120 to 140. High volume is a universal characteristic of effective training in every endurance sport. A second characteristic is a training-intensity distribution that is weighted heavily toward the low end of the intensity spectrum. Almost all endurance athletes do most of their training at lower intensities and a little at higher intensities. If a CTL of 120 to 140 is the magic number for maximum endurance performance, then this training-intensity distribution is to be expected. An athlete who does a large volume of high-intensity training will exceed the CTL range of 120 to 140 and burn out. An athlete who does most training at very high intensities will not be able to do enough volume to maintain a CTL higher than 120 without burning out because intensities above the lactate threshold are (literally) exponentially more stressful than intensities below the lactate threshold.

Most elites maintain **A PEAK CTL OF** **120–140** through **HIGH-VOLUME, LOW-INTENSITY TRAINING.**

Most endurance athletes cannot handle the volume of training required to maintain a CTL of 120 to 140 even if they do all of their training at low intensities. But the essence of the training approach that is proven to work best for elite athletes in all endurance sports (McGregor suspects that the 120–140 sweet spot applies in cross-country skiing and rowing too) works best for age-groupers as well. You will perform best and attain your racing weight quickest by maintaining a high training volume relative to your personal limits and by doing most of your training at lower intensities.

## HIGH VOLUME

Whatever you do—whether it's cycle, run, swim, or engage in all three—you need to do it a lot. How much? Train as much as you can without breaking down, burning out, or losing your job or spouse. If motivation is your limiter, then train as much as you can while still enjoying the training process.

The sheer amount of time you train has a stronger effect on your performance than any other factor. The reason has to do with efficiency. A low-volume, high-intensity approach to training will increase your aerobic capacity, or $VO_2max$, as much as a high-volume, low-intensity program. On a high-intensity program, however, you stop improving as soon as your $VO_2max$ hits a genetically defined ceiling, which doesn't take long. But with a high-volume program you become more and more efficient the longer you keep doing it, and so your race performances keep improving also.

The reason high volume yields ongoing efficiency gains is that each swim stroke, pedal stroke, and stride is an opportunity to practice that movement. The more you repeat it, the more practice you get, and the more practice you get, the more ways your neuromuscular system finds to trim waste from the movement pattern.

Exercise physiologist Edward Coyle performed physiological testing on Lance Armstrong from the time he started cycling professionally at age 20 until after he won his seventh Tour de France. During that period, Armstrong's $VO_2$max did not improve. But he most certainly improved as a cyclist, as evidenced by the fact that his best finish in his first four Tours was 36th place. Coyle's testing revealed that the physiological change that enabled Armstrong to elevate his performance long after his aerobic capacity was fully developed was an 8 percent improvement in his mechanical efficiency on the bike between the ages of 21 and 28. That came from years of consistent high volume. (Interestingly, efficiency is not affected by performance-enhancing drugs.)

A high-volume, low-intensity training approach is also a more effective way to shed excess body fat than a high-intensity, low-volume approach. It's a matter of simple math—and physiology. A 40-minute workout that includes five intervals of 4 minutes at 100 percent of $VO_2$max is a very hard workout. Few athletes would ever want to pack more training at such a high intensity into a single training session. The precise number of calories burned in this workout depends on the size of the athlete, the specific activity, and how much distance the athlete is able to cover. A 150-pound runner who covers 7 miles in this workout will burn about 787 calories.

Compare this to an easy 90-minute run covering 11.5 miles at 75 percent of $VO_2$max. This workout burns almost 1,300 calories, yet it is less stressful on the body than the shorter, faster run. This means the runner could do such runs a lot more often than he could do interval sessions and would thereby multiply the discrepancy in calorie burning.

## LOW INTENSITY

The question of the right approach to high-intensity training in endurance sports is controversial. Some coaches, trainers, and scientists advocate doing most training at high intensities with the understanding that the overall training volume must be kept low because the body cannot tolerate a high volume of high-intensity training. Others advocate a high-volume approach where most of the training is done at lower intensities and a relatively small amount of high-intensity training. Nobody champions a training approach that excludes high-intensity training, although some folks in the high-intensity camp like to argue against a straw man who does.

It is my observation that most representatives of the high-intensity camp come from backgrounds outside endurance sports, such as personal training and CrossFit, whereas all coaches of elite endurance athletes are squarely aligned with the low-intensity school. Among coaches of elite athletes there is consensus that most training should be done at lower intensities. This is not to say that there isn't some disagreement at this level. But the disagreement falls within narrow boundaries. An elite-level coach who considers himself a "volume guy" might have his athletes do 85 percent of their training below the lactate threshold and 15 percent at and above threshold. An elite-level coach who considers himself an "intensity guy" might have his athletes do 75 percent of their training below the lactate threshold and 25 percent at and above threshold.

The low-volume, high-intensity approach has been tried at the elite level of endurance sports. It was even the dominant model in some sports before the second half of the 20th century. But in the 1950s a New Zealand runner and coach named Arthur Lydiard experimented with a high-volume, low-intensity approach that soon transformed his tiny country into one of the world's top running powerhouses. Lydiard then took his approach to Finland, which became the next global running powerhouse. Runners everywhere began to copy the "Lydiard Method," and the high-intensity model was gradually abandoned at the elite level and has never returned. It was surpassed.

Exercise scientist Stephen Seiler and Finnish rowing coach Åke Fiskerstrand conducted a fascinating analysis of the evolution of training methods among world-class Finnish rowers between the 1970s and 1990s (Fiskerstrand and Seiler 2004). They learned that over that 30-year period average training volume had increased by 20 percent while high-intensity training volume had dropped by 33 percent. These changes were directly linked to improved performance. The best Finnish rowers of the 1990s pulled 10 percent more watts and consumed 10 percent more oxygen in standard rowing ergometer tests than had the best Finnish rowers of the 1970s.

The "modern" training intensity distribution of elite endurance athletes has been studied in various sports and places, and the results have been very consistent. A 1995 analysis of the training of national- and international-level swimmers over the course of a full season revealed that 77 percent of their swimming was done at or below a blood lactate level of 2 mmol/L, which is itself well below the lactate threshold level of 4 mmol/L (Mujika et al. 1995). And these were not distance swimmers but swimmers who specialized in the 100-meter and 200-meter sprints.

In 2001 Veronique Billat analyzed the training-intensity distribution of high-level French and Portuguese marathon runners (Billat et al. 2001). She discovered that these athletes did 78 percent of their training slower than marathon pace (which is slightly below threshold intensity for runners at this level) and 22 percent at marathon pace and faster.

Scientists who have conducted this type of analysis have developed a rule of thumb for training intensity distribution: the 80/20 rule. It stipulates that endurance athletes in all disciplines should aim to do roughly 80 percent of their training below the lactate threshold and 20 percent at and above threshold. (Some experts advocate an 80/10/10 rule, where 80 percent of training is below threshold, 10 percent is at threshold, and 10 percent is above threshold.)

**Train 80% below LACTATE THRESHOLD & 20% above.**

One could argue that the universality of the 80/20 training-intensity distribution among the world's best endurance athletes doesn't necessarily apply to nonelite athletes. After all, age-groupers do a fraction of the total volume that elites do. If they follow the 80/20 rule at such low volumes, they will do only a small amount of high-intensity work.

This is a sensible point, yet the best available evidence suggests that the 80/20 rule applies to nonelites as well. In a 2011 study researchers at the University of Stirling, Scotland, tracked the training of 10 age-group triathletes for six months as they prepared for an Ironman (Neal, Hunter, and Galloway 2011). The researchers calculated how much of the athletes' swimming, cycling, and running time was spent below lactate-threshold intensity, at threshold, and above. They also subjected the athletes to standard tests of swimming, cycling, and running fitness at the beginning and again at the end of the study period.

Remarkably, most of the subjects showed little improvement in fitness in any of the three disciplines despite six months of hard work. The reason might have been that they were working *too* hard. On average the athletes spent 30 percent of their total training time at or above the lactate threshold. In pushing themselves too often, the athletes were unable to fully absorb and adapt to their training. They started each workout a little tired and therefore got a lot less out of it than they should have.

An 80/20 training intensity distribution is appropriate for even the lowest training volumes. An example will drive home this point. A recreationally competitive runner with a busy life might run four times per week for a total of 3 hours. Here's what a typical week of training might look like for this runner if she followed the 80/20 guideline:

- **RUN #1:** 5 minutes easy warm-up; 9 x 2:00 at 3K race effort with 2:00 easy recovery jogs between intervals; 5 minutes easy cooldown
- **RUN #2:** 34 minutes easy
- **RUN #3:** 8 minutes easy warm-up; 18-minute "tempo" effort at 10K/10-mile race effort; 8 minutes easy cooldown
- **RUN #4:** 1 hour, 15 minutes easy

Runs #1 and #3 are not easy. As a supplement to the easy running in this schedule, they will supply this runner with enough of a challenge at faster speeds to elevate her racing performance. If there is a difference between the intensity distribution that's best for elite endurance athletes and the distribution that's best for recreational athletes, it's not that elites should do only 20 percent of their training at the lactate threshold and above while recreational athletes should do a higher percentage. Rather, the lowest-volume trainers should follow the 80/20 rule closely, while the highest-volume trainers may need to do less than 20 percent of their training at higher intensities.

Even though the proper place for high-intensity workouts in endurance sports training may be relatively small, it is extremely important. Numerous studies have shown that the addition of a small amount of high-intensity workout to a foundation of high-volume, low-intensity training quickly increases performance. For example, in one study researchers from Brigham Young University (Creer et al. 2004) separated 17 trained

> THE TIME DEVOTED TO HIGH-INTENSITY WORKOUTS IN ENDURANCE SPORTS TRAINING MAY BE RELATIVELY SMALL, BUT IT IS EXTREMELY IMPORTANT.

cyclists into two groups. One group performed only moderate-intensity training for four weeks. The other group included a very small amount of sprint training—just 28 minutes per week—in the training mix. Total work output increased significantly in members of the sprint group but not in the moderate-intensity group. Studies such as this one show that a little high-intensity training goes a long way to enhance performance through mechanisms that are complementary to those by which moderate-intensity training boosts performance.

The addition of a small amount of high-intensity training to a base of low-intensity training not only helps athletes take the last step toward peak fitness but also helps them take the last step toward their racing weight. In Chapter 3 I mentioned a study conducted by William Lunn at Southern Connecticut University. Cyclists either dieted, added high-intensity intervals to their training, or did both for 10 weeks. While the cyclists who added intervals without dieting did not lose weight, they did lower their already very low body fat percentage from an average of 10.1 to 9.9 through a small increase in muscle mass and a small decrease in fat mass.

## STRENGTH TRAINING

Strength training may be the last major innovation in endurance sports training. A generation ago most elite endurance athletes either did not do strength training, gave it lip service, or practiced primitive methods that have since been surpassed. Today strength training is taken very seriously at the elite level of every endurance sport. Even the runners of East Africa, most notably 27-time world record breaker Haile Gebrselassie, are starting to pump iron. The reason for strength training's spread through the elite ranks of endurance sports is its effectiveness. Strength training is proven to increase performance, reduce injury risk, and improve body composition in endurance athletes.

Some athletes who started their careers before the rise of strength training took it up in midcareer and reaped the benefits. In 2008, Dara

Torres, at age 41, attempted to qualify for her fifth U.S. Olympic swim team. To counteract the physical effects of aging, Torres incorporated an intensive dryland training regimen into her program. In the run-up to the Olympic Trials, she performed four 60-to-90-minute functional strength sessions per week with Florida Panthers strength-and-conditioning coach Andy O'Brien. The result was a chiseled physique, complete with six-pack abs (a rarity among swimmers) that drew a lot of attention during the Beijing Games. More importantly, Torres swam better than she had in her 30s, 20s, or teens, qualifying for the U.S. team in the 50-meter and 100-meter freestyle and winning silver medals in the 50-meter freestyle and two relay events.

If Torres is the poster girl of the strength training innovation in swimming, Michael Phelps is the poster boy. Between the 2004 and 2008 Olympics, Michael Phelps added five hours per week of strength training to his routine and successfully addressed the key weight-management challenge in swimming by adding 14 pounds of muscle—and a corresponding amount of strength and power—to his body.

The benefits of weight lifting on running performance were demonstrated in a 2008 study by Norwegian researchers (Støren et al. 2008). Seventeen well-trained runners were divided into two groups. Members of one group continued with their normal run training, while members of the other group added to their routine three weekly strength sessions consisting of four, four-repetition sets of half-squats using their four-repetition maximal load (i.e., the heaviest weight they could lift four times). After eight weeks, members of the strength group exhibited not only the expected gains in maximal strength and rate of force development, but also significant improvements in running economy (5 percent) and in time to exhaustion at maximal aerobic running speed (21.3 percent). The control group showed no improvement in any of the measured parameters.

How does lifting weights enhance running economy and endurance? Other studies have shown that it works by increasing the *stiffness* of the leg when the foot hits the ground (Dumke et al. 2010). The legs function as springs during running. Physics teaches us that a stiffer spring loses less energy when it lands and bounces higher. Your legs will do the same thing if you strengthen them in the gym.

It is worth noting that the loads used in this study were much heavier than those used by most endurance athletes in strength training. Endurance athletes are generally taught that they should use moderate loads and perform sets with large numbers of repetitions (12-rep sets are typical), because this approach imposes a strength-endurance challenge that is more relevant to endurance sports performance than the strength-power challenge imposed by lifting heavier loads. However, the point of hitting the gym if you're an endurance athlete is not to do the same type of training you do in your primary sport discipline(s). The point is to get a type of training stimulus that you are not getting from your endurance training. Lifting very heavy loads complements rather than merely reinforces their endurance training. And this Norwegian study proves it.

## LIFTING VERY HEAVY LOADS IS EXACTLY WHAT ENDURANCE ATHLETES SHOULD DO IN THE GYM BECAUSE IT COMPLEMENTS ENDURANCE TRAINING.

This is not to say that heavy lifting is the only sort of strength training endurance athletes should do. Core training exercises such as side planks do not entail lifting heavy loads, but they boost endurance performance by increasing joint stability and thereby removing waste from sports movements. This was demonstrated in a study performed by researchers at Barry University (Sato and Mokha 2009). Fourteen recreational and competitive runners participated in a six-week core strengthening program, before and after which their running kinematics, leg stability, and 5,000-meter running performance were tested. Another 14 runners served as controls by continuing to run during the six-week study period and not strengthening their core.

What did the researchers find in this case? Interestingly, core strength training was found not to affect the runners' ground reaction forces or leg stability (essentially balance on one leg), but it did improve their 5,000-meter race performance relative to members of the control group. The authors of the study did not speculate about why this effect was found. Based on my own research on the topic, I wouldn't be surprised to learn that it was mediated by an improvement in running economy resulting from more efficient transfer of forces between the upper body and the legs.

To get meaningful benefits from strength training, endurance athletes should perform strength workouts lasting 20 to 40 minutes apiece two to three times per week. You can accomplish much in a small amount of time with focused and efficient workout designs. Build your workouts from a mixture of exercises that increase your maximum strength and power in sport-specific movements and exercises that increase the stability of key joints in your sport, such as the shoulders if you are a swimmer. There is no need to pad your workout with multiple exercises for the same muscle group or numerous sets of each exercise. Just get in, go hard, and get out. The Appendix provides recommended strength exercises for various endurance sports.

Closely related to strength training is sport-specific power training, such as high-gear bike sprints and swimming kick sets with fins. Power training does not carry the injury-prevention benefit of strength training, but like strength training it improves performance and body composition.

The performance and body composition benefits of power training in cycling were demonstrated in a New Zealand study (Paton and Hopkins 2005). Researchers divided a team of cyclists into two groups. During an eight-week period within their competitive season, members of one group continued training normally, while members of a second group replaced two workouts each week with high-resistance, low-cadence strength intervals. All of the cyclists performed 40-km time trials before and after the study period. Over the eight weeks, members of the strength intervals group increased their mean time-trial power output by 7.8 percent compared to the control (or normally training) group. In addition, skinfold measurements suggested that the cyclists exposed to strength intervals lost a significant amount of body fat.

**INCLUDE 2-3 STRENGTH WORKOUTS LASTING 20–40 MIN. each week.**

As for maximum-intensity sport-specific strength and power development, even less is needed. I recommend that runners perform one set of 6–10 × 8–10-second sprints up a steep hill each week. Cyclists may perform either one set of 6–10 × 20-second power intervals (sprints in their highest gear) or steep hill sprints once per week. Since this type of training is difficult for cross-country skiers on actual snowfields, I recommend they use either the running or the cycling protocol just described, or both. Swimmers can and should spend

**TABLE 9.1 MAXIMUM-INTENSITY SPORT-SPECIFIC INTERVAL TRAINING**

| | FREQUENCY | EFFORT | SETS / DURATION |
|---|---|---|---|
| **Cyclists and cross-country skiers**/cycling | Weekly | Power intervals | 6–10 × 20 seconds in highest gear |
| **Rowers** | Weekly | Power strokes | 10–20 strokes at max effort |
| **Runners and cross-country skiers**/running | Weekly | Uphill sprints | 6–10 × 8–10 seconds |
| **Swimmers** | Weekly | Kicking sprints | 25 meters with fins on side |
| | Weekly | Pulling sprints | 25 meters with paddles |
| **Triathletes/cycling** | Biweekly | Power intervals | 6–10 × 20 seconds in highest gear |
| **Triathletes/running** | Biweekly | Uphill sprints | 6–10 × 8–10 seconds |
| **Triathletes/swimming** | 1–2x weekly | Kicking sprints | 25 meters with fins on side |
| | | Pulling sprints | 25 meters with paddles |

more time sprinting and developing power through kicking drills (e.g., sprint 25 yards on your side without using your arms while wearing fins; then flip over and repeat) and pulling drills (e.g., sprint 25 yards while wearing hand paddles), because such high-intensity work is less taxing in swimming and because pool swim races are short and require more strength and power. Triathletes should be training for strength and power in swimming, cycling, and running, of course, but they cannot do as much of each as single-sport athletes do lest they overwhelm themselves with the combination. I recommend that triathletes perform kicking and pulling drills once or twice a week in swimming and once every other week in cycling and running, on alternate weeks. In rowing, functional power is best developed with (what else?) power strokes: maximum-effort strokes of a specific count (usually 10–20) inserted into a longer, lower-intensity rowing effort.

With respect to strength training, then, athletes in every endurance sport should incorporate a bit of sport-specific strength and power training into their regimen—high-resistance sprints on the bike, steep uphill running sprints, and the like. These training modifications will not cause weight gain, but they will stimulate a slight increase in muscle mass that will in turn cause a proportional decline in fat mass by increasing fat burning after workouts and by elevating resting metabolism. Weight lifting and sport-specific strength and power training will also increase power by conditioning seldom-used fast-twitch muscle fibers and will reduce injury risk by improving the stability of the joints.

## Anabolic Eating

Gains in muscle strength and power cannot be maximized through training alone. Diet also contributes to muscular adaptations to strength and power training. If muscle strength and power are major concerns for you, then you will want to practice "anabolic eating" alongside your strength and power training. Anabolic eating is eating for muscle growth. While endurance athletes are not interested in muscle growth for its own sake, gains in muscle strength and power are closely linked to increases in muscle size. Use the following anabolic eating tips to get the most out of your strength and power training. Don't worry about "bulking up." There is absolutely zero chance that you will gain a burdensome amount of muscle weight through strength and power training and anabolic eating if you are also committed to a moderate- to high-volume endurance training program.

**MAINTAIN A CALORIC SURPLUS**. Research has shown that the most important dietary requirement for muscle growth is a caloric surplus. It is next to impossible to gain muscle mass if your body is burning more calories than it absorbs from food. This surplus need not be large, as muscle protein accretion is a slow process, and indeed your caloric surplus should not be large, as a large daily excess of energy intake will cause more fat storage than muscle gain. A surplus of 100 calories a day is plenty.

**EAT PLENTY OF PROTEIN**. Before you draw any conclusions about this advice, I should warn that it's not for the reason you think. It is widely believed that very high levels of protein intake are required to maximize muscle growth, but research has shown this belief to be false. A daily protein intake of 1.2 grams of protein per kilogram of body weight is sufficient to maximize muscle growth resulting from resistance training. While this level of protein intake is greater than the recommended minimum level of 0.8 grams per kilogram per day, it does not exceed the amount that the average person actually consumes. So there is no need to increase your level of protein intake to promote muscle growth.

However, increasing your protein consumption may help you minimize the body-fat gains that often accompany muscle growth. The reason is that dietary protein is less readily converted into body fat than dietary carbohydrate and fat. Consequently, if you maintain a diet with a 100-calorie daily surplus in which 30 percent of your calories come from protein, you are likely to gain less fat than if you maintain a diet with a 100-calorie daily surplus in which only 18 percent of your daily calories come from protein (which is average), although the amount of muscle gain is likely to be the same on both diets.

**EAT ANIMAL FOODS.** Animal proteins are more conducive to muscle growth than plant proteins, for a few reasons. First, they are "complete" proteins, meaning they contain all of the essential amino acids that the body cannot synthesize for itself, whereas proteins from plant foods are not complete. Second, animal proteins are more bioavailable than plant proteins, meaning they are more readily incorporated into the cells of the body. Only 78 percent of the protein contained in high-fiber legumes is actually digested, compared to 97 percent of the protein contained in animal foods. Finally, and not least important, animal foods tend to contain much larger amounts of protein than plant foods. For example, a large (1-cup) serving of brown rice contains only 4.5 grams of protein. By contrast, a small (3-ounce) serving of beef flank steak provides nearly 23 grams of protein.

For all of these reasons, you are likely to find it easier to gain muscle if you get most of your protein from animal foods such as fish and dairy products. However, it is certainly not impossible to gain muscle on a vegetarian diet. You just have to work a little harder at it. Because plant proteins are less bioavailable, you should aim for a target of 1.8 to 2.0 grams of protein per kilogram of body weight daily if you don't eat meat. Meeting this requirement will be much easier if you make regular use of vegetarian protein supplements such as soy protein shakes.

**EAT CARBS AND PROTEIN AFTER WORKOUTS.** The timing of protein consumption has a significant effect on the rate of muscle protein synthesis. Research has shown that protein consumed right before, during, and after exercise causes more muscle protein synthesis than equal amounts of protein consumed at other times.

The optimal amount of protein consumption after exercise is 20 grams. Consuming protein with carbohydrate after workouts is proven to result in even greater amounts of muscle protein synthesis. This is because carbohydrate stimulates the release of insulin, which in turn transports the amino acids from dietary protein to the muscle cells and initiates muscle protein synthesis.

**TAKE A CREATINE SUPPLEMENT.** Creatine phosphate is a fuel that the muscles rely on for maximum-intensity efforts such as sprinting 100 yards. Certain precursors of creatine phosphate, such as creatine monohydrate, are taken as supplements to increase creatine phosphate stores in the muscles. Research has shown that creatine supplementation enhances gains in muscle strength, size, and power resulting from resistance training, as well as performance in repeated high-intensity intervals. While creatine is extremely popular among strength athletes and recreational weight lifters, few endurance athletes use it. Yet it is likely to be helpful to those athletes who are seeking greater muscle strength and power.

# FOLLOW THE LEADERS

The nutritional and behavioral steps of the Racing Weight system that we explored in previous chapters—increasing diet quality, managing appetite, balancing the energy sources, monitoring performance, and timing nutrient intake—represent the tried and true weight-management methods of the most successful endurance athletes. As such, they should be emulated by all endurance athletes. The training step of the Racing Weight system is likewise an example set by the elites that nonelites must copy to reach their racing weight and realize their full performance potential.

If most age-group endurance athletes don't eat like the top professionals, even fewer train like them. I'm not talking about matching the volume that the pros put in. We mortals obviously cannot do that. I'm talking about emulating their winning approach, which entails prioritizing volume within your physical and psychological tolerance, keeping the intensity low most of the time yet going really hard when the time is right, and carving out a modest amount of time for strength training.

In my experience, and in that of many other coaches I've talked to, a majority of even the most competitive endurance athletes work out in a way that is the training equivalent of eating fast food three times a day—rushing through training sessions, getting workouts over with, steering clear of low and very high intensities like the gutters of a bowling lane, and giving lip service to strength training. The more you make your training regimen look like those of the men and women on the podium, the more your body will resemble theirs and the faster you will go when it really matters.

# FINE-TUNING YOUR STRATEGY

# PART III

# TEN

# THE RACING WEIGHT JOURNEY

T he Racing Weight system, which encompasses the six steps we've discussed in the preceding chapters, is not a diet program that you start on a particular day and stop several weeks later. Nor is it even a diet program that you start on one particular day and continue indefinitely. It is a set of tools that you use when you need them— namely, when you're trying to attain your racing weight for an upcoming race or series of races.

At other times you may not need these tools, or you may need a different set of tools. During breaks between performance-focused training cycles, it's not a bad idea to eat however you please for a couple of weeks. This will get any pent-up desire for low-quality foods and overindulgence "out of your system" so that you can get back on the Racing Weight system with renewed motivation when it's time to start training for your next race or races.

After your off-season break ends and before your next training cycle begins, you may choose to complete a four- to eight-week program for accelerated weight loss that I call a quick start. The purpose of a quick start is to shed excess body fat at a faster rate than you can within the training cycle, when performance is your top priority, through methods that are best kept outside the training cycle. The point of the quick start is not necessarily to take you all the way to your ideal weight and body composition but rather to get a quick start toward them. Any remaining excess body fat can come off more gradually on the Racing Weight system within the training cycle.

Quick starts are also appropriate for beginning endurance athletes who are significantly above their racing weight. An eight-week quick start will take these men and women down to a more comfortable weight at which to start training for their first race while also establishing a solid foundation of general fitness to build on. Beginners who are more than 20 pounds overweight may choose to extend their initial quick start beyond eight weeks. Theoretically, doing so would yield more weight loss in the athlete's first year or so in the sport than an eight-week quick start followed by a longer performance-focused training cycle.

However, in most cases I think it's best for beginners to hold their initial quick start to eight weeks and then get ready to race. After all, the goal of completing a race is more motivating than the goal of losing weight. Competitive goals encourage a higher level of dietary and exercise compliance than weight-loss goals, and therefore in the long term they produce better results.

It sometimes takes years for athletes who start their sporting journey overweight to attain their ideal racing weight. Few men and women who remain focused on weight loss as their primary goal have the patience to adhere to their program long enough to reach their destination. But

**TABLE 10.1 PLANNING YOUR RACING WEIGHT CYCLE**

| NUMBER OF CYCLES | JAN | FEB | MAR | APR | MAY | JUN |
|---|---|---|---|---|---|---|
| 1 | Preseason / QUICK START | | | PERFORMANCE | | |
| 2 | Preseason / QUICK START | | PERFORMANCE | | | Off-season |
| 3 | PERFORMANCE | | Off-season | Preseason / QUICK START | PERFORMANCE | |

those whose primary goal becomes improvement in their sport tend to stay consistent with their program because they are being rewarded—with better performance and its "side effect" of fat loss—every step of the way. I'll say more on this topic in the final section of this chapter.

# THE RACING WEIGHT CYCLE

Endurance athletes are accustomed to dividing the year into training phases. The central phase is the performance-focused training cycle, which starts when the athlete begins to seriously ramp up for a race or series of races and ends when this race or series is completed. The off-season is a period of relative rest between performance-focused training cycles. The preseason is a period of general preparation for the start of the next training cycle. In most endurance sports this is a period of heightened focus on strength development. Among cyclists and mountain bikers it is often also a period of aggressive weight dropping. For example, Jeremiah Bishop, winner of multiple national championships in mountain biking, maintains a daily energy deficit of 200 to 400 calories to drop weight before the start of a new racing season. He tries to keep his off-season weight gain to no more than 5–7 pounds because it takes a lot of work to get back to his racing weight, and that time would be better spent on quality training.

Because training and diet are synergistic, an endurance athlete's diet should have phases that match these three training phases. Within the training cycle the diet needs to support optimal training performance

| JUL | AUG | SEP | OCT | NOV | DEC | NUMBER OF CYCLES |
|---|---|---|---|---|---|---|
| PERFORMANCE | | | | Off-season | | 1 |
| Preseason / QUICK START | | PERFORMANCE | | | Off-season | 2 |
| Off-season | Preseason / QUICK START | PERFORMANCE | | Off-season | Preseason / QUICK START | 3 |

and facilitate the loss of excess body fat. In the off-season the athlete's dietary standards can be relaxed a bit, at least for the first two weeks. And during the preseason, or quick start period, the athlete eats to promote fat loss first and to support his or her training second.

Some endurance athletes will find that they cycle through these three phases once a year. An example is a cyclist who races from late spring through fall, takes a break for the holidays, and then starts preseason training after the New Year. Other athletes complete two cycles of all three phases. An example of this type is a runner who does a marathon in the spring and another in the fall with off-season breaks after each. Still others pack a trio of three-phase cycles into the year. An example of this type is a multidiscipline cyclist who does mostly road races in the summer, mountain bike events in the fall, and cyclocross competitions in the winter.

Table 10.1 summarizes the training and diet phases of athletes who complete one, two, or three full cycles in one year.

## THE TRAINING CYCLE

Regardless of how many racing weight cycles you complete within a year, you will practice the Racing Weight system the same way within each performance-focused training cycle. Each step is largely independent of the others, but when you're practicing all six together, they create a cohesive whole.

All of the steps allow and indeed require a degree of individualism in their execution. For example, daily carbohydrate requirements differ by body weight and training volume. There is also a natural evolution in some of the steps, such that they are not practiced in exactly the same way after a year or two as they are initially. For example, when you start to practice step 1, you will keep a daily food journal and calculate daily Diet Quality Scores as you seek to improve your diet quality. But once you've raised your diet quality to a level that works for you, daily food journaling and diet-quality scoring can be set aside as long as your diet remains consistent.

Here's a brief summary of how the six steps of the Racing Weight system are practiced together within the performance-focused training cycle:

1 **IMPROVE YOUR DIET QUALITY.** Start by keeping a daily food journal and calculating a daily DQS. Continue this as you make changes to your habitual eating patterns to increase your DQS. When your typical DQS is high enough to move you toward your racing weight, you may stop keeping a food journal and calculating your daily DQS, again provided your diet is consistent thereafter. Repeat this process whenever you make any significant change to your eating habits.

2 **MANAGE YOUR APPETITE.** Experience the difference between belly hunger and head hunger with a two-day appetite calibration. Thereafter use the mindful eating methods to satisfy your belly hunger only, and avoid additional, mindless eating from head hunger. All of these methods are optional. Find out which ones work best for you, and then stick with them.

3 **BALANCE YOUR ENERGY SOURCES.** Begin your first Racing Weight cycle by using Table 6.1 (page 102) to calculate your daily carbohydrate requirement. Next use the food journal you're already keeping for diet-quality scoring purposes to calculate how much carbohydrate you're actually consuming. Adjust your diet as necessary to meet your requirement. Recalculate your carbohydrate needs as your training load and body weight change.

4 **MONITOR YOUR PROGRESS.** Measure your body weight at least once a week and as often as once a day throughout each training cycle. Measure your body fat percentage at least once every four weeks and as often as once a week. Complete a sport-specific performance test once every four weeks.

5 **TIME YOUR NUTRIENTS.** Start eating breakfast every day if you don't already. Determine how many times a day you need to eat to avoid unacceptable levels of hunger at any point in the day and to support your training optimally. Once you've settled on a frequency that works for you—whether it's just three meals or three meals plus one to three snacks—stick with it until changes in your training load require you to add or eliminate snacking occasions. Establish habits of consuming fluid and carbs and perhaps also a little protein during your

more challenging workouts and of taking in recovery nutrition within 45 minutes of completing each workout.

6 **TRAIN FOR RACING WEIGHT.** Train by the 80/20 rule: Do approximately 80 percent of your training at lower intensities and 20 percent at and above the lactate threshold. Perform two to three full-body strength workouts per week.

# THE OFF-SEASON

A majority of elite endurance athletes I've surveyed on the topic of off-season diet tell me they eat less carefully during the off-season than they do within the training cycle. The rationale for such dietary slacking off is not physiological but rather psychological. Athletes find it easier to eat with great discipline within the training cycle when they give themselves an opportunity to reward that discipline between training cycles.

Weight gain tends to be unavoidable for many athletes in the off-season because of a reduction in training. When reduced training is combined with a slacker diet, the likelihood of weight gain is further increased. A small amount of off-season weight gain is not a bad thing. In fact it's a good thing inasmuch as it results from giving yourself a needed physical and mental break from the training and dietary rigors of the training cycle.

All too many endurance athletes gain too much fat in the off-season, however. Cyclist Jan Ullrich was infamous for letting himself go during the winter. His racing weight was 158 pounds, but he would routinely show up for his team's first training camp of the year at 180 pounds. He would perform poorly throughout the early season as he scrambled to work his body back into shape in time for July's Tour de France. Many cycling experts believe Ullrich would have won more than the one Tour he claimed at age 24 if he had taken better care of himself during the off-season.

Thanks to favorable genes, a few endurance athletes can slack off as much as they want in the off-season without putting on a whole bunch of fat (although not necessarily without losing a ton of fitness), but most endurance athletes, like most humans in general, have a built-in potential for rapid weight gain. The transition from peak-season training to off-season slacking presents the perfect circumstances for this potential to be unleashed.

The most effective way to prevent off-season weight gain from getting out of hand is to set a specific weight-gain limit. I suggest you try to limit your off-season weight gain to no more than 8 percent of your optimal performance weight. So if your optimal performance weight is 162 pounds, you should avoid gaining more than 13 pounds during the off-season. It so happens that my marathon racing weight is 154 pounds, and my off-season weight naturally peaks at 165 pounds (a difference of just over 7 percent) when I'm doing everything an endurance athlete should do in terms of training and nutrition at this time of year. But this 8 percent rule is not based only on my personal experience. It has been confirmed as a good rule of thumb by a number of other athletes, coaches, and sports nutritionists with whom I have discussed the topic of off-season weight gain.

Understand, however, that this rule is not an allowance to gain 8 percent of your end-of-season weight during the off-season regardless of what your end-of-season weight is. It is only an allowance to gain 8 percent relative to your optimal racing weight. If your weight is above optimum at the end of your competitive season, you should still limit your off-season weight gain to 8 percent relative to your (known or estimated) optimum. Thus, if you are already above your optimal racing weight at the end of the competitive season, you should try to avoid gaining any more weight during the off-season.

**LIMIT OFF-SEASON WEIGHT GAIN** *to* **<8%** *of optimal racing weight.*

The amount of weight you gain during the off-season depends on how much or little you train, how much your diet changes, and the length of your break. The last factor is likely to be determined by your future racing plans, which are completely up to you. Regardless of how long your off-season lasts, the initial period of zero training and eating whatever you want should last no longer than two weeks. After that you will need to reintroduce enough of the Racing Weight system to stay within 8 percent of your racing weight until you begin the next phase of the Racing Weight cycle: the quick start.

# THE QUICK START

The appropriate length of a quick start depends on how far above your racing weight you are when it begins. If you're less than 10 pounds above your racing weight, a four-week quick start will suffice. If you're between 10 and 20 pounds above your racing weight, a six-week quick start is best. If you're more than 20 pounds above your racing weight, try an eight-week quick start.

Whatever its length, your quick start is intended to yield faster weight loss than is possible within the training cycle, when building fitness is your top priority. Your nutrition and training practices in the quick start period are necessarily different from those in the performance cycle. There are five key dietary and training components of a quick start.

**STEP 1** **MODERATE CALORIE DEFICIT.** To lose weight, you must consume fewer calories than your body burns each day. In a quick start, your daily calorie deficit needs to be large enough to promote fairly rapid loss of excess body fat, yet not so large that you lack sufficient energy to perform well in your workouts. The calorie deficit "sweet spot" is 300 to 500 calories per day.

**STEP 2** **STRENGTH TRAINING.** During a quick start you should make a greater commitment to strength training than you do within the training cycle. Research has shown that when a calorie deficit is combined with strength training, nearly all of the resulting weight loss is actual fat loss. When a calorie deficit is not combined with strength training, weight loss is equal but body fat loss is less, because muscle mass is lost too. Building strength before you begin your performance-focused training will also give you a solid structural foundation to absorb that training.

**STEP 3** **INCREASED PROTEIN INTAKE.** While carbohydrate is king within the training cycle, I recommend that athletes switch to a high-protein diet—getting as much as 30 percent of their daily calories from protein—during the several weeks of a quick start. Protein is the most filling nutrient, and research has shown that "dieters" experience significantly less hunger when they combine a calorie deficit with increased protein intake. A high-protein diet will also help you get more out of your strength training.

**STEP 4** **FASTING WORKOUTS**. A fasting workout is a long, moderate-intensity workout undertaken in a fasting state—that is, without a meal beforehand and without carbohydrate consumption on the bike. When you deprive your muscles of carbohydrate in a long workout, they burn a lot more fat. Such workouts also boost general fat-burning capacity. I suggest that you perform one fasting workout per week during a quick start.

**STEP 5** **POWER INTERVALS**. Your training volume is necessarily lower during a quick start than it is during the performance-focused training cycle. You can't maintain maximum training volume year-round, or you'll burn out. Obviously, the higher your training volume is, the more calories you burn. So when your training volume is lower, as it is in a quick start, you need to burn calories in alternative ways.

Power interval sessions are one such alternative. These workouts consist of large numbers of very short intervals performed at maximum intensity (e.g., $20 \times 20$ seconds all out). Research has demonstrated that power intervals promote a high rate of fat burning in the hours that follow the session through a phenomenon known as EPOC (excess postexercise oxygen consumption).

**PUTTING IT ALL TOGETHER**. To complete a successful quick start, you must first determine exactly how many calories your body burns each day, because this provides the basis for setting your calorie deficit. You must then create meal plans that hit your daily calorie target and your 30 percent protein target simultaneously. You'll also need to design a sensible training plan that combines strength workouts, fasting workouts, and power intervals, plus the right amount of aerobic filler.

You can do all of this on your own, but I did it for you in the *Racing Weight Quick Start Guide*. This book presents complete four-, six-, and eight-week quick start plans that show you exactly how to eat and train to shed excess body fat rapidly and get a quick start on your next racing season.

# RACING FOR WEIGHT LOSS

Typically, endurance athletes manage their weight in order to perform better. They do not participate in endurance sports to lose weight. While endurance activities such as running are excellent ways to lose weight, those men and women who take up such activities primarily to lose weight seldom stick with them. An American College of Sports Medicine study (Havenar and Lochbaum 2007) of individuals participating in a group training program for first-time marathoners found that those whose primary motivation was weight loss were significantly more likely to drop out than were those whose primary motivation was to achieve event-related goals.

Overwhelmingly, the men and women who stick with an endurance activity long enough to become full-fledged endurance athletes cite simple enjoyment of the activity as their primary motivator for pursuing it. In a companion study to the Montana State University study on endurance athletes' weight-related beliefs, attitudes, and practices mentioned in the Introduction, respondents were asked to select their top three reasons for exercising from a list of ten options. Enjoyment ranked number one. Weight loss ranked dead last (Stults-Kolehmainen et al. 2009).

The poster child for these principles is Natascha Badmann, a six-time winner of the Hawaii Ironman. In her early 20s, Badmann, who is Swiss, was an overweight and depressed single mother who loathed the very idea of exercise. A coworker at her office (Badmann was employed as a secretary at a computer company) noticed Badmann nibbling on tiny lunches at noon and then gorging on chocolate later in the day. He kindly explained to her that if she wanted to lose weight, she needed to eat more lunch and less chocolate and that she needed to exercise.

Although she had no interest in working out, Badmann was determined to lose weight, and she thought her coworker, Tony Hausler (now her husband), was kind of cute, so she accepted his offer to take her running and cycling. In the beginning she could not even run a mile, and she suffered through every step. A triathlete, Hausler understood the psychology of exercise and thus steered Badmann's attention away from weight loss and toward developing competence and enjoying a feeling of accomplishment on the bike and on her two feet.

Hausler talked Badmann into participating in a short duathlon only six months after she started training with him. Upon crossing the finish line, she was hooked. And it did not hurt that, thanks to her one-in-a-million endurance genes, she took 3rd place.

Duathlon, and later triathlon, gave Badmann a sense of identity and purpose and made her feel good about herself. Endurance sports also made her lose weight, but after a few months she had lost all the weight she needed to lose, and maintaining her losses was the last motivation to keep going. Five years after completing her first half-mile run, Badmann became the duathlon world champion, and a year after that she took 2nd place behind the legendary Paula Newby-Fraser in the Hawaii Ironman.

Affectionately nicknamed the "Swiss Miss," Badmann is a favorite of triathlon fans because she wears a smile throughout every race, win or lose. What started as a reluctant means to weight loss has become for her a source of the greatest happiness.

So that's the fairy-tale version of the phenomenon. But there are millions of less extreme cases that are no less meaningful in the lives of everyday folks. Consider the case of Wesley Howarth, an IT professional from Liverpool, England. Wes had been a competitive Olympic weight lifter in his youth, but he downshifted from competitive to recreational training at age 17 and then let himself go altogether in his early 30s. At age 35 he was hospitalized for three months with a condition that was eventually diagnosed as chronic myofascial pain. His weight ballooned to 342 pounds.

One day after his release from the hospital, Wes stepped on a scale, and it registered an error message because his weight exceeded its measurement capacity.

"I decided to change my life right then," he says.

Wes had always hated aerobic exercise but knew he had to bite the bullet and do it to lose weight. He was so out of shape that he began with 10-minute walks. But while he couldn't exercise long, he could exercise often and consistently, and by doing so, he was able to make rapid progress, advancing from longer walks to walk-jog workouts to real running. And as he made progress, something magical happened: He started to enjoy running.

Inevitably, Wes began participating in races. His first event was a 5K. He has since moved up to half-marathons and marathons. Wes's headlong leap into endurance sports has resulted in a most welcome and unexpected side effect: He no longer has to take medication for his once burdensome pain condition. He's also lost 124 pounds and hopes to lose 20 more. However, "weight loss has become secondary," he says. It's pure enjoyment that keeps Wes running (and swimming, biking, and strength training). "As much as I used to hate running, that's how much I love it now," Wes confirms.

Beginning endurance athletes often need to change their mind-set before they can fully enjoy the many benefits (including weight loss) of staying involved in their sport over the long term. Too often, they are motivated primarily by a goal to lose weight. Ironically, they will lose more weight if they replace this goal with performance goals and with a focus on simply "getting hooked" on their new sport. Enjoyment and the desire to perform better are the only motivations that can keep endurance athletes involved in their sport, and loss of motivation is the greatest barrier that prevents beginning endurance athletes from getting lean and light and enjoying the other benefits their sport offers. So if you are new to endurance sports, I want to give you some additional guidance to help you build and maintain motivation to participate in your sport.

## GUIDELINES FOR BEGINNERS

Endurance training is an acquired taste. Learning to love an endurance sport involves learning to love physical straining, extreme fatigue, and sore muscles. Granted, pain and suffering may not be what endurance athletes love most about training and racing, but these two results are inseparable from the greatest joys of training and racing, such as the joy of getting faster. So it's not surprising that most passionate adult endurance athletes first fell in love with exercise as children, when the physical straining of exercise was introduced as play.

In this regard my story is utterly typical. I took up running at age 11 after watching my dad run the Boston Marathon. He never told me to run or even encouraged me to run. He just ran and enjoyed it, so I thought I might enjoy it too. I did not seek weight loss, fitness, approval, glory, or any other reward from running—just enjoyment. And enjoy it I did.

I wish every child could be so fortunate as to experience an early, positive introduction to exercise. Yet while the story of my early affinity for exercise may be the norm, and while it may be easiest to develop a passion for endurance sports as a youth, previously exercise-averse adults catch the endurance bug every day.

## SUCCESSFUL BEGINNERS SHOULD FOCUS ON PERFORMANCE AND ENJOYMENT OVER WEIGHT LOSS.

I meet such folks all the time in the course of my work. For example, on a flight to Bermuda to cover the Escape to Bermuda Triathlon, I met Bryan Lee, a 46-year-old furniture store owner from Seattle, Washington. In conversing with Bryan over the Atlantic Ocean, I learned that he had taken up triathlon the previous spring, having been a nonexerciser his whole life. It started when a cousin, who happened to be a Navy SEAL, invited Bryan to his wedding, and Bryan decided to try to get in shape so that he did not make his cousin "look bad" at the big event. (Bryan was roughly 40 pounds above his college weight.) So he joined a triathlon training class, confident that all the swimming, cycling, and running involved would quickly trim him down and tone him up, but having no intention of actually completing a triathlon ("because those people are crazy," he recalled thinking).

Unexpectedly, Bryan discovered that he actually liked the class, and he signed up to participate in a local sprint triathlon after all. Self-admittedly obsessive-compulsive, he developed an instant endorphin addiction, began looking for races to do every weekend, and was soon traveling all over the world (Chile, South Africa, Monaco, and so forth) for fixes. Escape to Bermuda was to be his 35th triathlon in 18 months. He had lost 35 pounds along the way, but losing weight had long since ceased to be his main motivator for swimming, cycling, and running. "I just love the whole lifestyle," he said.

Bryan Lee's story contains some important cues about how best to develop a love for endurance sports, which should be every beginning endurance athlete's first objective. Weight loss can be a goal as well—indeed, if you need to lose weight, it should be a goal—but understand that you are unlikely to still be exercising one year from now if you don't learn to enjoy your training.

There are four key steps in the process of learning to enjoy exercise.

## CHOOSE A SPORT THAT FEELS RIGHT

In our society exercise is promoted as a means to achieve desired results rather than as an end in itself. Exercise product manufacturers and service providers compete by promising better results through more efficient means. Advertisers assume that you cannot possibly enjoy exercise; therefore fitness solutions are marketed on claims of minimizing the amount of time the consumer is required to suffer through them to achieve the results he or she wants. This phenomenon is epitomized in the best-selling fitness book *8 Minutes in the Morning*, which promises a body like that of author Jorge Cruise, with a commitment to exercise not exceeding the eight minutes of the title, and in the infomercials for the Bowflex exercise machine, which promise bodies like those of the fitness models they show using the machine "in just minutes a day."

Such marketing encourages consumers to choose modes of exercise utterly without regard for any possible affinity for the activities themselves. It teaches us to view working out strictly as a chore to get through as quickly as possible and hence to choose the particular form of exercise that will yield the desired results in the least amount of time. But there is no form of exercise that yields the results we really want in just minutes a day. It takes hours a week, every week, to sculpt and maintain a fitness model's body, and it is nearly impossible to sustain that level of commitment unless exercise is enjoyable.

Despite such efforts to make us believe that some forms of exercise are more effective than others, the truth is that all forms of exercise are more or less equally effective—if you keep doing them. But you're unlikely to keep doing any form of exercise that you view as a chore to be gotten over with as quickly as possible. Only if you truly enjoy the actual experience of performing a given form of exercise can it become a permanent part of your lifestyle.

So if there's a particular endurance sports activity that you've tried in the past and kind of liked, make it your primary form of exercise going forward. If you haven't yet found a favorite, try them all and choose the one that feels most "right" as you do it.

## SET A BIG GOAL

I encourage every beginning endurance athlete to set his or her sights on finishing a race. Establishing such a "big" initial goal seems counterintuitive to many, but it's actually a much surer way to cultivate enjoyment of exercise than setting a small goal, such as losing 10 pounds. The reason is that big goals are more consonant with human psychology.

First, any goal tends to be most motivating when it is quite challenging. Small, easy-to-achieve goals don't always excite or, frankly, frighten us enough to inspire consistent hard work toward their fulfillment. Setting a goal to finish a first race—whether it's a sprint triathlon, a century ride, a half-marathon, or something else—will make exercise a "bigger deal" in your daily life and encourage you to invest more in it, thereby accelerating the process of coming to enjoy it.

Second, research in psychology has shown that human beings are natural game players. Almost any sort of hard work becomes more enjoyable when it is structured as a game, with a clear objective and clear means of "counting points" or measuring progress toward that goal. When I was a child, my mother cleverly made a game of the chore of putting away my toys before bedtime—a chore that my two brothers and I loathed. She would put a fun song on the record player and challenge us to put all of our toys away before it ended. We raced around giggling and screaming instead of moping and pouting as we had always done when tidying up in the past. More to the point, studies in exercise psychology have demonstrated that men, women, and children have more fun playing sports than they do exerting themselves at the same intensity in mere fitness activities (Bakshi, Bhambhani, and Madill 1991). By establishing a goal to finish a race, you transform an activity, such as bicycling, that could be a mere fitness activity into a sport.

Third, research has also shown that self-efficacy, or a feeling of activity-specific competence, is the single best predictor of enjoyment in a given activity, and pursuing and achieving the goal of completing a race are a great way to develop a sense of self-efficacy in your chosen endurance sport (Lewis et al. 2002). The first distance-running race I ever completed was a roughly 1-mile run against my fellow fifth-graders on our school's annual field day. It hurt like hell, but I won, and the winning made me want to race again, despite the suffering that racing entailed. Studies in sports and exercise psychology indicate that my experience was quite typical. The naturally fittest kids (and adults, for that matter) tend to most enjoy fitness activities, while the naturally most coordinated kids and adults most enjoy motor skill sports, such as basketball. In short, we most enjoy doing what we do well.

Does this mean you have to be capable of winning races to enjoy an endurance sport? Fortunately, it does not. Research suggests that exercise enjoyment increases as fitness does. Thus, as long as you enjoy your chosen sport well enough to continue doing it until you get that first race under your belt, you will gain so much fitness and self-efficacy along the way that you will enjoy it much more by the time you have achieved that initial goal. Also, crossing your first finish line has a magical effect on self-efficacy. It's transformative in many cases, such as that of furniture salesman–turned–triathlete Bryan Lee. Something about stopping the clock at the end of an official event puts a hook in you, such that no sooner have you showered off your race sweat than you are already plotting your next race goal.

## GO OVERBOARD

A change of lifestyle is a big deal because it is also a change of identity. Your self-definition is transformed in the process of making significant modifications to your daily routines and rituals. Because major lifestyle changes are often disruptive, they are not completed without a certain rallying of your entire personality around the change. This is why a honeymoon period of intense absorption in a new lifestyle often occurs. We see the phenomenon played out in every sphere of life. Perhaps you know someone who found religion as an adult and couldn't stop talking about God for a while. You can probably think of at least one person who found a career and threw himself into it headlong, suddenly dressing the way people in that profession dress, talking the way they talk, and so forth.

The same pattern is normal in endurance sports. Running, triathlon, or whatever it is becomes the biggest thing in the beginner's life for a time as she develops a new sense of identity as an athlete that is essential to learning to enjoy sport and establish it as a permanent lifestyle component. Bryan Lee is once again an extreme case in point, completing 35 triathlons in his first 18 months as a triathlete. He'll want to slow down sooner or later, of course, as he will need to be balanced in the long run. But in the novice endurance athlete, a short-term imbalance in the direction of obsession with the new hobby is normal and healthy.

I am not quite instructing you to become obsessed with your newly chosen endurance sport, because such a thing cannot be forced. Either it happens on its own, or it doesn't happen at all. I will only advise you that should obsession begin, do not try to stop this process through misguided self-doubt, conscience, or sense of propriety. If you find yourself feeling compelled to read all the books and magazines on your sport, pass time on related Web sites, purchase new gear every week, seek out new friends in your sport, and so forth, let it happen. Go ahead. Go overboard!

## REMOVE BARRIERS

If you are not currently a regular exerciser, then there are barriers between you and exercise. They are the very reasons you have not exercised consistently to this point. As such, these barriers, which may be logistical, psychological, social, and perhaps even physical in nature, must be dismantled if you are to succeed in becoming a bona fide endurance athlete who enjoys exercise.

The primary logistical barrier to exercise is time. Lack of time is the most commonly cited excuse for not exercising. But surveys suggest that those who exercise regularly are just as busy with their jobs, families, and other responsibilities as those who don't work out. So the time excuse is just that: an excuse. We're all pressed for time, yet we all have time for our highest priorities. If exercise is important to you, you will find the time to do it. Consider the case of David Morken, an age-group triathlete whom I had the pleasure of profiling for Ironman.com a few years ago. Morken is a husband, an involved father of six children, and the CEO of a high-tech company, and yet still he finds enough time to train for triathlons. If David Morken can do it, anybody can!

Creative ways that endurance athletes find to fit training into their schedules include working out early in the morning and late in the evening, commuting to and from work on foot or by bicycle, working out on their lunch break, packing most of their training into weekends, working out indoors at home (for example, cycling on an indoor trainer), and combining workouts with other responsibilities (for example, running laps around a soccer field while your child's team practices on it). You might be amazed to see how creative you become after you drop the time excuse!

Perhaps the greatest psychological barriers to exercise, after lack of exercise enjoyment itself, are lack of self-esteem and the attending demons of self-doubt, pessimism, and fear of failure. Lifelong nonexercisers are often ashamed of their bodies and convinced they cannot accomplish anything positive with them. There are many effective methods of battling these internal barriers. Recognizing that they exist is the first. Once you recognize that your expectation of failure in exercise is a self-fulfilling symptom of low self-esteem, instead of a rational deduction based on solid evidence, it will suddenly seem worthwhile to make every effort to destroy this illusion. Other methods to employ in this effort include seeking your family's support and encouragement, exercising with a friend or a group of like-minded individuals, speaking encouragement to yourself (possibly in the form of inspirational notes left in key locations, such as on your car steering wheel), and even seeking professional counseling if you feel you could benefit from it. Remember, you really are worth every effort made to learn to enjoy exercise and become an endurance athlete (who just happens to be lean and look great)!

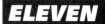

# ELEVEN

# RACING WEIGHT FOODS

very person's diet has staple foods—foods that are eaten frequently for their taste, nutrition, or convenience. While it is good to have variety in your diet, there's nothing wrong with relying on staple foods as long as they are healthy. In fact, eating staple foods can be an effective way to maintain consistency in your diet, and consistency is proven to be helpful in weight management.

Some foods work especially well as staples for endurance athletes who are working toward their racing weight. Twenty-six of these foods will be presented in this chapter. You could attain your racing weight with a completely different set of staples. But these 26 foods appear again and again in the food journals of the world's best endurance athletes, so you can't go wrong with them.

Whichever foods you choose as staples, be sure to eat a variety of them. Your body will not be as well nourished as it ought to be if 80 percent of your calories come from only half a dozen foods. But the real opportunity to include healthful variety in your diet lies outside of the staples. If, say, 75 percent of your calories are regularly accounted for by a dozen staple foods, the other 25 percent should come from a much longer and indeed ever-changing list of foods.

I've organized the suggested staples by food category. There are six foods from the vegetable category, five from the fruit category, five from the lean meats and fish category, four from the nuts and seeds category, four from the whole grains category, and three from the dairy category.

Healthiness is not the only important quality in a staple food. You won't see a lot of exotic foods in my list. I believe that by and large the best staple foods for endurance athletes are simple foods that are a familiar part of the cultural diet. The Racing Weight foods are easy to get, relatively affordable, and universally enjoyed. It makes sense to draw Racing Weight foods from the foods that are readily available (with a few exceptions).

Many of the Racing Weight foods can be eaten as they are; many others can be prepared very simply. Some are available in healthy packaged products and restaurant menu items. Of course, if you like to cook or enjoy gourmet home-cooked meals, you can get as fancy as you like with these foods. To prime your imagination, I've included several recipes containing Racing Weight foods that were created especially for this book by Pip Taylor, a world-class triathlete, nutritionist, and chef from Australia.

# VEGETABLES

The word "superfood" is used in reference to plant foods that have special health-enhancing properties. In fact, every vegetable is a superfood. But in my opinion these six are particularly super for endurance athletes.

## BEETS AND BEET JUICE

Beets are a flavorful, versatile vegetable with a very high concentration of a class of antioxidants known as betalains. Research has shown that betalains have uniquely powerful anti-inflammatory properties, so they help athletes with postworkout recovery.

Beet juice is even more beneficial for athletes. It contains a high concentration of nitrates, which help the blood vessels dilate during exercise, increasing blood flow to the working muscles. Studies have shown that drinking beet juice significantly enhances endurance performance (Cermak, Gibala, and van Loon 2012). Try drinking 750 ml of beet juice two hours before important workouts and races for a performance boost.

## VEGETABLE SOUP

Vegetable soups are a hot counterpart to smoothies. Whereas smoothies are a tasty and convenient way to get a big dose of fruit, vegetable soups are a yummy and expedient way to get a big dose of veggies. To make one, you need do no more than puree your chosen vegetable (potato, sweet potato, white beans), mix in some water and spices, and bring the whole thing to a boil. There are also some very good canned vegetable soups that are even easier to prepare. One of the most nutritious vegetable soups is good old-fashioned pea soup. Peas are a good source of carbohydrate and are also rich in vitamins A, C, B6, and K as well as folate, magnesium, phosphorous, and fiber.

Vegetable soups are excellent Racing Weight foods because they fill the stomach without a lot of calories. Eating a small bowl of soup at the start of a meal is an effective appetite-control technique.

## SPINACH

Spinach is one of the most nutritionally complete foods that nature has to offer, boasting a "Completeness Score" of 93 on nutritiondata.com's 1–100 scale of nutritional balance. The vegetable's versatility and familiarity make it a terrific staple food. Many endurance athletes eat raw spinach in salads, eat cooked spinach in dishes such as Pip Taylor's Goat Feta, Spinach, and Potato Frittata, and even add spinach to smoothies because it blends well and allows fruit flavors to dominate.

## SWEET POTATO

Sweet potatoes are trendy these days—so trendy that you can get sweet potato french fries at many fast-food restaurants. That's not how you should include these nutrient-rich vegetables in your diet, however. Baked, grilled, and mashed sweet potatoes are much less calorie dense, and even some recipes for sweet potato pie and homemade sweet potato wedges are acceptable.

Sweet potatoes are rich in carbohydrate, fiber, and antioxidants and were once rated the most nutritious vegetable by the Center for Science in the Public Interest. They make a great Racing Weight staple because they are one of the most satiating high-carbohydrate foods.

# Goat Feta, Spinach, and Potato Frittata

*Frittatas make a quick breakfast, lunch, or even dinner when served with a simple green salad. They can be eaten hot, at room temperature, or cold, so you can prepare them in advance easily. Any variations of ingredients can be used; try combinations of mushroom, ham, tomato, and roasted pumpkin—even cooked pasta can be added.*

4  lb. potatoes, skin on
Olive oil spray
½ of a small onion, thinly sliced
1  cup baby spinach leaves, washed and dried

Sea salt and pepper to taste
4  large eggs, lightly beaten
2½ oz. goat feta cheese (low fat), crumbled

1. Preheat an oven broiler/grill to high. Meanwhile, cook potatoes until tender either in boiling water for several minutes or covered in the microwave. Slice into ½-inch-thick slices and set aside.
2. Heat a nonstick ovenproof frying pan over medium heat, and spray with a small amount of olive oil. Add onion and cook for 2–3 minutes, stirring until soft and starting to turn golden. Add potato slices and spinach and toss gently, adding salt and pepper to taste. Pour eggs over the mixture, stir gently from the edges of the pan inward for 30 seconds, and then crumble goat cheese over the top.
3. Allow the mixture to cook over low/medium heat for 5–6 minutes until nearly set. Turn off the heat and place pan under a hot grill for 2–3 minutes until frittata is puffed and golden.
4. Let sit in pan for about 5 minutes, and then slide out onto a cutting board and slice into wedges.

**NUTRITIONAL FACTS PER SERVING (daily value)**

CALORIES 384, TOTAL FAT 20 g (31%), SATURATED FAT 9 g (43%), CARBOHYDRATE 30 g (10%), FIBER 4 g (18%), SUGARS 5 g, PROTEIN 21 g (42%), CALCIUM 261 mg (26%), CHOLESTEROL 454 mg (151%), IRON 3 mg (19%)

## HEIRLOOM TOMATOES

Tomatoes are technically a fruit, but I prefer to go with culinary, rather than botanical, convention and classify them as a vegetable. Regardless of how you classify them, tomatoes just aren't what they used to be. It's so hard to find a good tomato these days that most people under the age of forty have no idea what a good one is. If you ever do eat a really good tomato, you can bet that it's an heirloom—a tomato grown from seeds that have not been hybridized for better appearance and shelf life (at the cost of less taste). If you can find a reliable source for heirloom tomatoes, do yourself a favor and pay extra for them. If you can't find them locally, buy seeds and grow your own.

Like other tomatoes, heirlooms are celebrated for their dense content of lycopene and other antioxidants. Regular tomato eaters have a lower risk of heart disease, perhaps because of those antioxidants. Heirloom tomatoes are a good friend to athletes pursuing their racing weight because they add a lot of flavor to foods without adding a lot of calories.

I drink tomato juice almost every day with my lunch and wish every endurance athlete did. Substituting tomato juice for whatever you normally drink with your lunch is a very easy way to increase your diet quality. Although it's not made with heirlooms (and it includes beets, spinach, and other vegetables in addition to tomatoes), Spicy Hot V8 juice is my personal favorite.

## AVOCADOS

It's hard to believe that health-conscious eaters used to avoid avocados for their high fat content. Now everyone knows that the unsaturated fats in avocados are good for the body. Avocados (which are in season at different times, depending on where they grow) also contain a rich assortment of other nutrients.

One of the reasons avocados are designated as a Racing Weight food is that they make a good substitute for fattening condiments. A burrito with guacamole doesn't need sour cream; a sandwich with avocado can do without mayonnaise.

# Fish Tacos with Avocado, Tomato, and Corn Salsa

*A deceptive variety of nutrition is delivered in this delectably simple lunch recipe.*

2  7-oz. firm white fish fillets such as snapper or blue eye, cut into three strips
1  tsp. olive oil
1  tsp. paprika
1  tsp. ground cumin
1  cup fresh corn kernels (or canned corn, drained)
2  small tomatoes, chopped roughly

1  small red chili, chopped fine
1  lime, juiced, plus extra lime wedges to serve (optional)
1  tsp. fresh coriander leaves (cilantro), finely chopped
Sea salt and black pepper
1  avocado, chopped
4  small, soft, wheat-tortilla wraps

1. In a shallow dish, combine olive oil, paprika, and cumin and mix into a paste. Add fish strips and turn gently to coat. Set aside while you prepare the salsa.
2. Combine corn (if using fresh corn, cut the kernels from the cob and then cook in boiling water for 2 minutes) and tomatoes with chili, lime juice, and chopped coriander. Add chopped avocado, season to taste with salt and pepper, and mix gently.
3. Heat a frying pan to a medium-high heat. Add fish to pan and cook for 2–3 minutes (depending on thickness of fish); then turn and cook a further 1–2 minutes.
4. Meanwhile, heat tortillas by wrapping them in foil and placing them in oven on low temperature or by wrapping them in a paper towel and microwaving for 30 seconds (or according to package instructions).
5. Place warm tortilla on a plate, and top with strips of fish and salsa. Serve two tacos per person with lime wedges.

**NUTRITIONAL FACTS PER SERVING (daily value)**

CALORIES 635, TOTAL FAT 25 g (38%), SATURATED FAT 4 g (20%), CARBOHYDRATE 63 g (21%), DIETARY FIBER 13 g (52%), SUGARS 7 g, PROTEIN 46 g (92%), CALCIUM 159 mg (16%), CHOLESTEROL 86 mg (29%), IRON 5 mg (30%)

# FRUITS

Most fruits are seasonal, ripening in either the spring, summer, fall, or winter. Fruits taste best and are most nutritious when consumed in season. Those grown out of season in hothouses are no match nutritionally. They're still high-quality foods that will help you attain your racing weight, but I recommend that you eat the following Racing Weight fruits in season as much as possible.

## APPLES

The high fiber and water content of apples make them highly satiating. This characteristic and their portability qualify apples, an autumn fruit, as terrific Racing Weight snack foods. Apple-based desserts like Pip Taylor's Baked Apple, Cranberry, and Maple Pudding are higher-quality desserts than most other desserts, such as ice cream and cookies.

## BANANAS

In the past decade or so bananas have become an underappreciated food because they have a lower antioxidant content than many other fruits. Overall, though, bananas are as nourishing as any other fruit. They are packed with vitamins and minerals, have a high fiber content, and are a terrific source of carbohydrate.

I designate bananas as a Racing Weight food because they are a natural alternative to ergogenic products such as energy bars and carbohydrate gels. Their high carbohydrate content (27 grams in a medium-sized fruit) and ease of consumption and digestion them make them an ideal preworkout and pre-race food.

Bananas are also beneficial during exercise. In a 2012 study published in the online journal *PLoS One*, 14 trained cyclists completed a pair of 75-km time trials, eating bananas during one of them and drinking a sports drink during the other (Nieman et al. 2012). The two energy sources were rationed to ensure that the subjects took in the same amount of carbohydrate in both time trials.

The average finish time was about three minutes, or 2 percent, faster in the sports drink time trial than in the banana time trial. The difference, however, did not meet the minimum threshold for statistical significance, so the Appalachian State University scientists who conducted the study concluded that the effects of the two energy sources on performance were equal.

# Baked Apple, Cranberry, and Maple Pudding

*If you prefer, substitute pears or even mixed berries for the apples in this recipe.*

4 apples, peeled, cored, and quartered

2 medium eggs

1 cup whole milk

⅓ cup pure maple syrup (or golden syrup)

½ cup all-purpose flour

1 tsp. cinnamon

¼ cup dried cranberries

1 tsp. butter

1. Preheat oven to 350°F. Cut each apple quarter in half. Then cut each piece crosswise into four parts so that you are left with small chunks.
2. In a bowl, lightly whisk the eggs with the milk and maple syrup. Add the flour and cinnamon and whisk until just combined, stir in the apple and cranberries, and set aside.
3. Use butter to lightly grease a medium-sized shallow baking dish. Pour apple mixture into the dish, and bake in the oven for about 30 minutes until set, puffed, and golden.

**NUTRITIONAL FACTS PER SERVING (daily value)**

CALORIES 284, TOTAL FAT 5 g (7%), SATURATED FAT 2 g (9%), CARBOHYDRATE 56 g (19%), DIETARY FIBER 3 g (11%), SUGARS 37 g, PROTEIN 7 g (14%), CALCIUM 121 mg (12%), CHOLESTEROL 111 mg (37%), IRON 2 mg (10%)

## CHERRIES

Cherries are one of the best fruits for endurance athletes. A spring fruit, they are rich in antioxidants that have strong anti-inflammatory effects in the body. Studies have shown that drinking tart cherry juice reduces exercise-induced muscle damage and postworkout muscle soreness. Eating whole cherries will have the same effect.

My wife and I have a cherry tree in our backyard, so we are acutely aware of how brief the cherry harvest is. But dried cherries are almost as nutritious (the fruit loses some of its antioxidants when it's dehydrated) and delectable, and they are available year-round.

## ORANGES AND ORANGE JUICE

Orange juice is already a staple in the diets of many endurance athletes, as it is in the diets of nonathletes. It's a worthy staple too, supplying lots of carbs, vitamin C, and antioxidants including hesperidin, which improves blood vessel function. While more exotic fruit juices such as pomegranate and açaí are all the rage these days, orange juice is just as good and generally a lot cheaper. The best staples typically are healthy foods that are well ingrained in the cultural diet, and orange juice is one such food.

Have you ever wondered why orange juice is a traditional breakfast beverage? It started about 100 years ago when the orange industry responded to an orange glut by creating a marketing campaign that encouraged Americans to start their morning by "drinking an orange." Although the custom is arbitrary, I encourage athletes to just go with it because most traditional breakfast foods do not contain fruit. Better yet, use orange juice in a Breakfast Smoothie like Pip Taylor's.

Even more nutritious than orange juice is the whole orange, a winter fruit. One large orange contains 4 grams of fiber, which are missing in the juice.

**SERVES 1**

# Breakfast Smoothie

*An on-the-go breakfast alternative. The almond butter adds protein and essential fats to help you feel and stay full.*

1 banana
½ cup blueberries (frozen are best in this recipe)

½ cup plain yogurt
½ cup milk or orange juice
1 Tbsp. almond butter

**1.** Blend all ingredients and drink.

### NUTRITIONAL FACTS PER SERVING (daily value)

CALORIES 389, TOTAL FAT 17 g (26%), SATURATED FAT 7 g (33%), CARBOHYDRATE 52 g (17%), DIETARY FIBER 6 g (23%), SUGARS 35 g, PROTEIN 14 g (28%), CALCIUM 303 mg (30%), CHOLESTEROL 28 mg (9%), IRON 1 mg (5%)

## RED GRAPES (AND RED WINE)

Among the many healthy phytonutrients in red grapes is one called resveratrol, which is not only healthful but also beneficial to endurance performance. Animal studies have shown that resveratrol supplementation increases aerobic capacity by enhancing heart function and muscle force production. The doses of resveratrol used in these studies have been much greater than those supplied by red grapes, but a little is undoubtedly better than none, and grapes have a lot else going for them besides resveratrol, including a high fiber content.

Red wine lacks the fiber of whole red grapes, but it has the resveratrol. Studies have demonstrated that drinking red wine regularly in moderation significantly reduces the risk of heart disease. The alcohol content of red wine is believed to be partly responsible for this effect because moderate consumption of all types of alcoholic beverages is known to boost heart health. So rather than include either red grapes or red wine in your diet, why not include both?

# LEAN MEATS AND FISH

There are dozens of varieties of meat and fish that are worthy of being classified as Racing Weight foods. But these five are especially worthy.

## FARMED TROUT

Trout is one type of fish that is better to buy from a farmed source because wild lake trout often contains higher levels of toxins. Rainbow trout is a relatively lean fish with only 8 grams of fat per fillet. Like all fish, it is rich in high-quality protein to help your muscles recover from and adapt to training.

A tender table fish with a slightly sweet flavor, rainbow trout is often enjoyed even by those who do not consider themselves fish lovers. You don't have to be a gourmet chef to prepare a delicious trout recipe. Try pan-frying a couple of fillets and flavoring them with pepper and lemon juice, and then go from there.

## GRASS-FED BEEF

Beef is one of the food world's best sources of protein and of creatine, a compound that fuels maximum-intensity muscular efforts. Beef from grass-fed cattle is an even better protein source and also has less total

# Stir-Fried Beef and Mushrooms with Snow Peas and Hokkien Noodles

*Stir-fries can be varied depending on what is at hand and what is in season. Chop the vegetables relatively thin and roughly the same size so that they cook in the same amount of time. Experiment with different sauces by adding chili or ginger, and try different types of noodles. Although this recipe calls for the use of Hokkien noodles, which are traditional rice noodles used in Southeast Asian stir-fries, any type of rice noodle will do.*

½ lb. Hokkien noodles or any other Asian egg-based noodle
8 shitake mushrooms, dried
½ Tbsp. peanut oil
¾ lb. lean beef, such as top sirloin, cut into strips
1 small onion, sliced thin
2 cloves garlic, crushed
1 cup snow peas, with strings removed
1 Tbsp. oyster sauce
1 Tbsp. soy sauce
1 Tbsp. rice wine
1 tsp. sesame oil

1. Place Hokkien noodles in a large bowl and cover with boiling water (following package instructions). Let stand; then separate noodles gently and drain. Rinse with cold water; then drain again and set aside.

2. Meanwhile, place dried mushrooms in a small bowl, cover with boiling water, and set aside for 5 minutes. Drain (reserve mushroom water to use as stock in another recipe, such as a risotto). Remove stems from mushrooms and discard; then slice caps.

3. Heat peanut oil in a wok (or large frying pan) over high heat. Stir-fry beef in two batches until browned (about 3–5 minutes), and then remove. Add onion to wok and cook until golden. Then return meat to pan along with garlic, snow peas, mushrooms, oyster sauce, soy sauce, and rice wine. Cook for an additional 3 minutes. Then add noodles and sesame oil.

4. Toss well until noodles are heated through. Serve immediately.

**NUTRITIONAL FACTS PER SERVING (daily value)**

CALORIES **823**, TOTAL FAT **44 g (68%)**, SATURATED FAT **8 g (41%)**, CARBOHYDRATE **83 g (28%)**, DIETARY FIBER **5 g (21%)**, SUGARS **4 g**, PROTEIN **43 g (86%)**, CALCIUM **96 mg (10%)**, CHOLESTEROL **83 mg (28%)**, IRON **8 mg (42%)**

fat, more essential fatty acids, and a lower calorie density that its grain-fed counterpart.

As a staple of the American diet, beef is plentiful, relatively inexpensive, familiar, and broadly enjoyed. So it's easy to make beef a staple in a Racing Weight diet as well. But most of the beef that Americans eat comes in fast-food hamburgers and tacos. You don't want that. Make lean cuts of grass-fed beef your staple instead.

## TUNA

Tuna is the world's most popular table fish. It is also very nutritious and is therefore a well-qualified food staple for endurance athletes. Some varieties of tuna, including albacore and bluefin, are rich in omega-3 fatty acids. As we saw in Chapter 6, these essential fats have special benefits that go beyond their basic health benefits. They reduce exercise-related free radical damage to the muscles, improve reflexes, and increase cardiac efficiency.

Canned tuna can be—but isn't always—as good as the fresh tuna that is used in sushi and tuna steaks. Some canned tuna products are high in mercury and relatively low in omega-3 fats, and some contain added oils that greatly increase their calorie density. Among the best brands of canned tuna are High Seas, Island Trollers, and Wild Planet.

## TURKEY BREAST

The popularity of turkey as a deli meat soared when concerns about fat in the diet steered Americans away from bologna and ham. Today turkey sandwiches are probably the most popular sandwich choice among healthy eaters, including endurance athletes. And an excellent choice they are. Leaner cuts of turkey breast are almost completely fat free and, of course, are an excellent source of protein.

Why limit turkey breast to lunches, though? As a man who would probably choose a traditional Thanksgiving dinner as his last meal, I believe that the association of turkey with that holiday results in an unfortunate turkey avoidance in dinner menus the rest of the year. Seriously, though, it is a shame, because turkey dinners are wonderful and there's no better protein to include in your dinner. So start carving up some turkeys in July to help your body absorb the heavy training you're doing then.

# Tuna Mac 'n' Cheese

*Mac 'n' cheese that is good for you! Once you've mastered this recipe, try using roasted pumpkin and peas, or even add chopped cherry tomatoes, asparagus, or broccoli.*

1 lb. dried short pasta such as macaroni, penne, etc.
½ Tbsp. olive oil
2 cloves garlic, crushed
1 small onion, finely chopped
1 large zucchini, grated
1 large carrot, grated
6.5-oz. can corn, drained

15 oz. evaporated skim milk
1 Tbsp. cornstarch
½ cup water
6.5-oz. can water-packed tuna, drained
5 oz. low-fat cheddar cheese, grated
½ cup dried breadcrumbs

1. Preheat oven to 350°F. Cook pasta according to package instructions, drain, rinse under cold water, and drain again before setting aside.
2. Meanwhile, heat a large nonstick frying pan over medium heat. Add the olive oil, then add garlic and onion, and sauté until translucent. Add zucchini, carrot, and corn and cook a further minute. Then add evaporated milk. Bring mixture to a slow simmer while stirring.
3. In a small glass bowl, combine cornstarch and water and mix to dissolve. Then add to the pan, stirring continuously. Cook a further 2 minutes, bringing back to simmer until the mixture thickens. Turn off heat.
4. Return pasta to the pot, and add in the sauce mixture, tuna, and 3.5 oz. of the grated cheese. Mix well. Spoon into a large baking dish. Combine the remaining cheese and breadcrumbs, and sprinkle over the top.
5. Bake for about 30 minutes until the topping is crunchy and bubbly.

*Note:* This dish can be prepared the night before and stored covered in the refrigerator. In that case, it will just take a little longer in the oven (about 40 minutes) to heat all the way through.

**NUTRITIONAL FACTS PER SERVING**

CALORIES **682**, TOTAL FAT **6 g (9%)**, SATURATED FAT **2 g (9%)**, CARBOHYDRATE **118 g (39%)**, DIETARY FIBER **7 g (29%)**, SUGARS **13 g**, PROTEIN **38 g (77%)**, CALCIUM **232 mg (23%)**, CHOLESTEROL **22 mg (7%)**, IRON **3 mg (18%)**

## WILD SALMON

Wild salmon is more expensive and harder to obtain than farmed salmon but is preferable because it has significantly lower levels of PCBs and other toxins. Both wild and farmed salmon are excellent sources of omega-3 fats.

To get enough essential fats in your diet, you need to eat fish at least twice a week or take a daily essential fatty acid supplement. Even if you do take a supplement, it's beneficial to include fish in the diet since regular fish eaters tend to be leaner than those who avoid fish. With its unique taste and texture, salmon is one of the most widely appealing table fish and has thus become a top seafood staple. If you eat fish, make it a staple in your Racing Weight diet.

# NUTS AND SEEDS

It's not necessary to get a large fraction of your total calories from nuts and seeds, but it is good to eat this category of foods frequently. I suggest that you eat these four Racing Weight nuts and seeds most often.

## CHIA SEEDS

Chia seeds are the edible seeds of a plant that is native to Central and South America. They are often called a superfood because of their well-balanced nutrition. Chia seeds contain protein, omega-3 essential fats, fiber, and minerals. They can be eaten raw, soaked in water to create a beverage known as chia fresca, blended into smoothies, and ground for use in baking. Sprouted chia seeds are similar to alfalfa sprouts and are worthy additions to sandwiches and salads.

While they are not a traditional staple of the American diet, chia seeds are becoming increasingly popular among endurance athletes, and with good reason.

## HEMP SEEDS

Hemp seeds share the balanced nutrition and versatility of chia seeds. Three tablespoons of shelled hemp seeds provide 11 grams of high-quality protein, 11.4 grams of omega fatty acids, 1 gram of fiber, and lots of iron, zinc, phosphorous, and magnesium.

You can eat hemp seeds raw, but most people prefer to add hemp seed meal to hot and cold breakfast cereals, smoothies, and baked goods. Sprouted hemp seeds are great in salads and sandwiches.

Like chia seeds, hemp seeds are on their way to becoming a staple seed food among endurance athletes in the know.

## OLD-FASHIONED PEANUT BUTTER

Read the nutrition label to make sure your peanut butter is simply peanuts and salt. Although peanuts are technically a legume, they are called nuts because they have much in common with actual nuts nutritionally. They are especially rich in heart-healthy monounsaturated fats. Regular peanut and peanut butter eaters are less likely to develop cardiovascular disease, in part because of the fats these foods contain but also because of their high antioxidant content, which rivals that of strawberries.

My favorite way to consume peanuts is in peanut butter, a traditional American lunch and snack staple whose healthier versions (products containing only peanuts and salt) are also great staples in the diets of endurance athletes. While calorically dense, peanut butter is highly satiating, so it aids appetite management. Spread peanut butter on toast in the morning, use it in a sandwich at lunchtime, or dip carrots into it as an afternoon snack. Some athletes even use peanut butter in smoothies (it goes well with bananas, coconut milk, and spinach).

Peanut allergy is among the most common food allergies. If you have it, you know it and you avoid peanuts. For everyone else, peanuts are purely good.

## ROASTED CASHEWS

If you're looking to stave off midmorning or midafternoon hunger and at the same time boost your diet quality by eating foods in the nuts and seeds category, there's no easier way to check both items than eating a handful of roasted cashews. Few foods offer a more even balance of macronutrients—1 ounce of cashews contains 9 grams of carbohydrate for muscle fuel, 5 grams of protein for muscle rebuilding, and 12 grams of mostly unsaturated fats for appetite control.

# WHOLE GRAINS

If you make these four whole grains staples in your diet, you will seldom have to eat lower-quality refined grains.

## BARLEY

A close relative of wheat, barley has a nuttier flavor and, when cooked, a more chewy consistency than its more popular cousin. Like all whole grains, barley is an excellent source of carbohydrate (44 grams per cup) and fiber (6 grams per cup). This combination makes it an excellent Racing Weight food because it provides precious muscle fuel in a highly satiating package.

A versatile food, barley can be mixed with wheat flour in baking; added to hot cereals, soups, and stews; and used in pilafs and risottos like Pip Taylor's Pearl Barley Risotto with Shrimp, Lemon, and Baby Spinach. Barley is also a key ingredient in many beers, which, when consumed in moderation, are healthy in the same way that wine is.

## BROWN RICE

Brown rice has become the most accessible whole grain next to whole wheat. Restaurants such as the Mexican food chain Chipotle offer brown rice as an alternative to white rice in menu items, and packaged food makers such as Minute offer precooked brown rice products that can be prepared in 10 minutes or less. Brown rice's accessibility, high carbohydrate content (45 grams per cup), and fiber richness (4 grams per cup) make it a top Racing Weight food.

## OATS

Old-fashioned oatmeal is one of the best breakfasts for endurance athletes, especially when the diet quality of the meal is bolstered with the addition of fresh fruit, dried fruit, nuts, seeds, and/or milk. A popular and traditional breakfast food, oatmeal supplies the body with a substantial amount of carbohydrate in a form that is easy to digest. Whole oats may also be used in other workout- and race-powering breakfast cereals such as Pip Taylor's Bircher Muesli.

In the general population oats improve insulin sensitivity, stabilize blood glucose, prevent free radical damage, enhance the immune response to infection, and inhibit weight gain. All of these health

# Pearl Barley Risotto with Shrimp, Lemon, and Baby Spinach

*Pearl barley gives this risotto a slightly different flavor than is found in traditional recipes, while spinach makes it more nutrient dense.*

½ Tbsp. olive oil

1 small onion, finely chopped

2 cloves garlic, peeled and minced

1½ cups pearl barley, rinsed under cold water and drained

2 cups chicken stock

2 cups water

½ lb. raw shrimp, peeled and deveined

1 Tbsp. lemon zest

2 cups baby spinach leaves

1 Tbsp. fresh parsley, finely chopped

1 Tbsp. fresh basil, finely chopped

1. Set a large, heavy-base saucepan or pot on medium heat, and cook the olive oil, onion, and garlic until soft and translucent. Add the pearl barley and stir until it is coated with the onion mixture.

2. Add the stock and cook, stirring until the liquid is absorbed (about 10–15 minutes); then add the water and continue to cook, stirring frequently until the liquid is absorbed and the barley is tender but still al dente (firm to the bite). This will be about 30–35 minutes of total cooking time.

3. Add the shrimp, lemon zest, and baby spinach and stir. The shrimp will take only several minutes to change color and be cooked through. Stir in the herbs and season to taste.

*Note:* If you don't have time to stand at the stove and stir the risotto, it can also be baked in the oven. After sautéing the onion and garlic on the stove top, add the pearl barley and the liquid (stock and water), and then bake in a preheated oven at 350°F for 30–35 minutes until liquid is absorbed and barley is tender to the bite. Remove from oven, stir in shrimp, lemon zest, and spinach, and return to oven for 5–10 minutes until shrimp is pink and just cooked through.

**NUTRITIONAL FACTS PER SERVING (daily value)**

CALORIES 800, TOTAL FAT 10 g (16%), SATURATED FAT 2 g (10%), CARBOHYDRATE 135 g (45%), DIETARY FIBER 25 g (101%), SUGARS 8 g, PROTEIN 45 g (91%), CALCIUM 167 mg (17%), CHOLESTEROL 177 mg (59%), IRON 8 mg (45%)

# Bircher Muesli

*This is a very simple version of soaked, bircher-style muesli. Oats are soaked overnight, and the rest of the ingredients are stirred through in the morning. Alternatively, if you forget to do this the night before, add ¼ cup of water to the oats along with berries (if using frozen) and microwave on high for 30 seconds before stirring in the yogurt and chopped apple. Substitute your favorite seasonal fresh fruits and nuts to mix things up.*

¾  cup rolled oats
½  cup plain yogurt
1   cup mixed berries
    (raspberries, blueberries,
    etc., frozen or fresh)

1   apple, cored and chopped
    (leave skin on)
1   Tbsp. raw nuts (almonds,
    macadamias, walnuts, etc.)

1. The night before, combine oats, yogurt, and berries if you are using frozen ones. Leave covered in the refrigerator.
2. In the morning, stir in chopped apple and berries if you are using fresh, and then top with nuts.

**NUTRITIONAL FACTS PER SERVING (daily value)**

CALORIES 452, TOTAL FAT 8 g (13%), SATURATED FAT 3 g (17%), CARBOHYDRATE 121 g (40%), DIETARY FIBER 11 g (44%), SUGARS 47 g, PROTEIN 15 g (31%), CALCIUM 195 mg (19%), CHOLESTEROL 16 mg (5%), IRON 4 mg (24%)

benefits, which come partly from the high antioxidant content of oats, carry over to sport. Increased insulin sensitivity, for example, enables the muscles to take up nutrients faster during exercise and during recovery after exercise.

## WHOLE WHEAT

Whole wheat's reputation has been besmirched in recent years by the gluten-free diet trend. It is true that a tiny fraction of the population—namely, persons with celiac disease—cannot eat wheat because they cannot tolerate its gluten protein content, and perhaps another 1 percent of the population is better off not eating wheat because of sensitivity to gluten or other proteins in wheat. But a large and growing number of people who tolerate wheat perfectly well are eating wheat-free or gluten-free diets because they believe that gluten and wheat are simply "bad." This is not true. If you're among the 98 percent of people who do not experience nausea, abdominal cramping, and other symptoms, then there is no need for you to avoid wheat.

In fact, if you're an endurance athlete, there is more than one reason to include whole wheat in your diet. It is the most accessible whole grain in the American diet, found in all kinds of breads and other baked goods as well as in breakfast cereals. Like other whole grains, it provides substantial amounts of carbohydrate and fiber to fuel the muscles and manage appetite.

# DAIRY

A tremendous variety of foods are made from milk. Some are better for endurance athletes than others. These three are especially good.

### FETA CHEESE

Traditionally made not with cow's milk but with sheep's or goat's milk, feta cheese is a crumbly, salty cheese popular in Greek cuisine. Because it has a strong flavor, feta is typically used in small amounts in salads and vegetable dishes. Such meals are among the healthiest and least-calorie-dense ways to incorporate dairy in the diet.

### PLAIN YOGURT

As I mentioned in Chapter 4, a Harvard University study found that yogurt prevented long-term weight gain more effectively than any other food, including fruits and vegetables. This study did not distinguish varieties of yogurt, but the best Racing Weight yogurt is plain yogurt (either traditional or Greek) without added sugar. Add your own fruit to it, or add it to cereal-and-fruit mixes or smoothies such as Pip Taylor's Breakfast Smoothie (page 187).

### WHOLE MILK

Most health-conscious eaters assume that reduced-fat milk is healthier than whole milk because the latter has a high saturated fat content. However, most studies comparing the health effects of whole milk and

# Zucchini, Mint, and Feta Filo Pies

*These are quick to make—most of the required time goes toward waiting for them to bake. Try other vegetables such as cooked spinach, chopped asparagus, green peas, corn, cherry and sun-dried tomatoes. Makes eight pies.*

4  small zucchinis, grated
½ small onion, finely chopped
4  medium eggs, lightly beaten
3½ oz. feta cheese, crumbled
⅓ cup fresh mint, chopped fine
Salt and pepper to taste

8  sheets filo pastry (found
   in the freezer section)
Oil spray
Premium-quality tomato
   chutney to serve (optional)
Salad leaves to serve (optional)

1. Preheat oven to 350°F. Put grated zucchini into a strainer and push gently to remove some excess water, then put into a mixing bowl. Add onion, eggs, feta, and mint leaves and mix, then season to taste. Set aside as you prepare the pie cases.

2. Try to work quickly once the filo pastry is opened so that it does not dry out. You can buy a little extra time by covering it with a dry tea towel topped with a damp cloth. Place filo in a pile so that there are eight layers on top of each other. Cut into eight pieces approximately 4 inches square. Spray eight holes of a regular-size muffin tin lightly with oil, then take two layers of filo and push down into each hole. Spray the pastry lightly, then place another two layers of filo on top, positioning them at right angles so that the whole of the muffin hole is covered. They will look a little rough and wrinkly.

3. Spoon zucchini mixture into cases until they are two-thirds full. Do not overfill as they will puff slightly as they bake and may overflow.

4. Cook in oven for 30–35 minutes until set and golden brown. Let sit for about 15 minutes. Serve warm or at room temperature with chutney and salad.

5. Leftovers can be stored in an airtight container in the refrigerator.

**NUTRITIONAL FACTS PER SERVING (daily value)**

CALORIES 288, TOTAL FAT 13 g (20%), SATURATED FAT 6 g (29%), CARBOHYDRATE 30 g (30%), DIETARY FIBER 4 g (14%), SUGARS 5 g, PROTEIN 14 g (29%), CALCIUM 196 mg (20%), CHOLESTEROL 208 mg (69%), IRON 4 mg (21%)

reduced-fat milk have identified no differences, while a majority of studies that have identified differences have given the advantage to whole milk. For example, a nine-year epidemiological study involving nearly 20,000 middle-age women reported that whole-milk drinkers were slightly leaner than skim-milk drinkers (Rosell, Håkansson, and Wolk 2006). The reason may be that whole milk is rich in conjugated linoleic acid, which promotes muscle growth and fat loss.

Beyond these advantages, whole milk is less processed than reduced-fat milk. As a general principle it is best to consume all foods in their least-processed forms. What's more, whole milk tastes better. If you regularly use whole milk, even 2% milk tastes like water in comparison.

Few people drink milk of any variety anymore. I'm old enough to have grown up drinking milk, as most children once did. I stopped drinking milk when I reached adulthood, and I won't ask you to start. But I do recommend that you add whole milk to breakfast cereals, coffee drinks, smoothies, and whatever else you normally add milk to.

# WHAT THE PROS EAT

The Racing Weight system is based on the weight-management practices of the best endurance athletes. The six steps that the highest-performing athletes most often take to attain their racing weight are by definition the most effective weight-management methods for endurance athletes because the objective of weight management in endurance sports is better performance. The surest way to reach your racing weight is to simply copy these practices.

Copying the weight-management methods of the best athletes is not the same thing as eating exactly what they eat. There is a lot of variety in the diets of top endurance athletes because following one specific diet is not among the six weight-management steps that these athletes practice. These steps leave plenty of room for individual choices. For example, while a large majority of world-class endurance athletes maintain high diet quality, there are dozens of ways to maintain a high-quality diet.

While eating exactly what the pros eat is not what the Racing Weight system is all about, it is instructive to know exactly what they do eat. Studying the specific food choices of the highest-performing cyclists, rowers, runners, skiers, swimmers, and triathletes helps other athletes appreciate what is required and what is allowable in the successful pursuit of racing weight. For example, you will see a lot more vegetables than sweets in the food journals of the best endurance athletes—proof that a high-quality diet is required. But you won't see many named diets (Paleo, Zone, gluten free, etc.) at this level—proof that all food types and a variety of ways of eating are allowable in the pursuit of racing weight.

In order to help you better appreciate what it takes (and what it doesn't) to attain racing weight, I have gathered a selection of one-day food journals from a handful of the highest-performing athletes in a variety of endurance disciplines. If you see one or more specific choices that you would like to copy, go for it, but do not feel obligated to do so. It's not the exact foods but the general methods of improving diet quality, managing appetite, balancing energy sources, monitoring performance, timing nutrients, and training for racing weight that you must emulate.

# JEREMIAH BISHOP

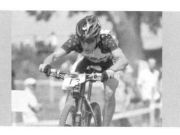

Jeremiah Bishop is a professional MOUNTAIN BIKER with the Cannondale team. Based in Harrisonburg, Virginia, Bishop is the winner of multiple national championships in marathon and short-track cross-country racing. Despite his high fitness level and clean diet, Bishop has high blood pressure owing to genetic inheritance, which he is able to control without medication. The following one-day food journal is from an early-season training period when Bishop was intentionally eating 200 to 400 fewer calories than his body burned daily.

**BREAKFAST**

1 cup oatmeal with raisins and cranberries

Optygen HP (herbal supplement)

2 cups coffee

2 tsp. flax oil

1 shot MonaVie Active (açai juice supplement)

**WORKOUT** *(ride)*

2 bottles Cytomax sports drink

1 bottle water

2 Cytomax gels

1 PowerBar

**POSTWORKOUT**

Cytomax recovery drink

**LUNCH**

Italian wedding soup

Turkey sandwich with provolone

Small mixed green salad with carrots and cherry tomatoes

Fresca

**AFTERNOON SNACK**

Fig Newman cookies

Raw Revolution bar

Black tea

**DINNER**

Large mixed green salad with smoked salmon, grated Parmesan cheese, tomatoes, carrots, olives, mandarin ginger dressing

MonaVie Pulse red yeast rice (for treating high cholesterol)

Bio 35 multivitamin

# MEGAN KALMOE

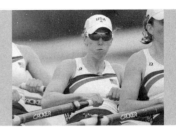

Megan Kalmoe is a ROWER who won a bronze medal in the 2012 Olympic quadruple sculls event. The previous year she won a silver medal in the same event at the World Rowing Championships. Kalmoe placed 1st with Ellen Tomek in the 2008 U.S. Olympic Trials Women's Double Sculls and was a 2005 under-23 world champion in the Women's Four. Here's how she eats during the peak summer training period.

**BREAKFAST**

1 cup bran flakes with
½ cup organic skim milk,
¼ cup blueberries

1 cup orange juice
(not from concentrate)

1 whole wheat English muffin
with 1 Tbsp. Smart Balance butter
spread, 2 Tbsp. raspberry jam

8 oz. regular drip coffee, black

**WORKOUT 1** *(rowing)*

20 oz. Gatorade (from powder mix)

32 oz. water

1 GU packet (if doing anaerobic
threshold or power work)

**POSTWORKOUT**

1 CLIF bar

1 banana

8 oz. coffee

**MORNING SNACK**

2 whole eggs, scrambled

2 slices whole wheat toast with
1 Tbsp. Smart Balance spread

8 oz. orange juice

**LUNCH**

1 serving leftover homemade
lasagna made with regular pasta,
part-skim ricotta, part-skim
mozzarella, zucchini, ground turkey

1½ cups raw carrots with
¼ cup hummus

12 oz. brewed iced tea

**AFTERNOON SNACK**

1 medium apple with 2 Tbsp. chunky peanut butter

2 white cheddar rice cakes

**WORKOUT 2** *(rowing)*

20 oz. Gatorade (from powder)

20 oz. water

**DINNER**

5 slices homemade pizza made with homemade white dough, homemade tomato sauce, part-skim mozzarella, fresh homegrown basil, vine-ripened tomatoes, fresh whole garlic

Small green salad with cucumber, carrot, onion, sunflower seeds, 1½ Tbsp. raspberry-walnut salad dressing

12 oz. seltzer water

1 slice angel food cake with ½ cup homemade blueberry sauce (blueberries, sugar, lemon juice)

8 oz. water

# RYAN HALL

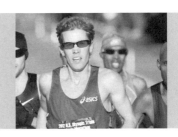

Ryan Hall is a **RUNNER** who is the American record holder in the half-marathon (59:43) and the fastest American-born marathoner of all time (2:04:58). The food diary below was recorded a couple of weeks after Hall finished 3rd in the 2009 Boston Marathon, when he was staying at the Olympic Training Center in Chula Vista, California, "where they provide some pretty incredibly tasty and healthy eats," he said. "I usually don't eat this gourmet at home." (Note: Ryan drinks 20 oz. water when he wakes up every day.)

**BREAKFAST**

1 cup Trader Joe's Flax Crunch cereal with Cytomax recovery shake (1 scoop) substituted for milk

1 Tbsp. Trader Joe's sunflower seed butter

**WORKOUT 1** *(run plus calisthenics)*

Lots of water

**POSTWORKOUT**

1 slice sourdough bread with 1 Tbsp. almond butter

**LUNCH**

4–6 oz. steak

4–6 oz. polenta with sautéed mushrooms and onions

2–4 oz. orzo with feta and spinach

2 cups steamed veggies (broccoli, cauliflower, zucchini, yellow squash, carrots)

**AFTERNOON SNACK**

2 slices sourdough bread with sunflower seed butter

**WORKOUT 2** *(bike ride, gym workout, self-massage)*

Water

**DINNER**

Spinach salad with grape tomatoes, green and red peppers, mushrooms, cottage cheese, Caesar dressing

4 oz. pork with ½ cup applesauce

1 cup steamed broccoli

¾ cup chipotle polenta

1 slice French bread

½ cup pasta

½ cup baked beans

**EVENING SNACK**

Handful of trail mix

# KIKKAN RANDALL

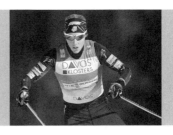

Kikkan Randall is an elite **CROSS-COUNTRY SKIER** who lives in Anchorage, Alaska. She represented the United States in the 2002, 2006, and 2010 Winter Olympics. In 2009 she won a World Championships silver medal in the sprint event, and in 2012 she was the World Cup overall sprint champion. A 10-time high school state champion runner in Alaska, Randall took up skiing to keep fit for track and cross country. Now she runs to keep fit for skiing and she still races on foot occasionally, winning the 2011 Mount Marathon in Seward, Alaska. Here's what Kikkan eats on a typical day of summer training.

## BREAKFAST

1 egg, ½ cup pure egg whites,
2 Tbsp. shredded cheddar cheese

2 slices Canadian bacon

2 slices whole wheat toast with
2 Tbsp. raspberry jam

4 oz. orange juice

8 oz. tea with skim milk, sugar

**WORKOUT 1** *(skate rollerskiing)*
24–32 oz. PowerBar
Endurance sports drink

## POSTWORKOUT

20 oz. PowerBar Recovery drink

6 oz. fat-free yogurt

1 medium banana

## LUNCH

6-in. Subway sandwich made
with turkey, pepper jack cheese,
veggies, honey mustard on
wheat bread

1 small bag Baked Lays
potato chips

12 oz. lemonade

1 macadamia-nut cookie with
white chocolate chips

## AFTERNOON SNACK

1 cup Frosted Mini-Wheats cereal

⅔ cup skim milk

1 skim mozzarella cheese stick

**WORKOUT 2** *(skate rollerskiing)*
24–32 oz. PowerBar
Endurance sports drink

## POSTWORKOUT

20 oz. PowerBar Recovery drink

2 slices whole wheat bread
with 2 Tbsp. peanut butter,
1 Tbsp. honey

## DINNER

Steak fajitas made with 3 oz.
marinated steak, 1 cup kidney
beans, 1 cup cooked onions and
bell peppers, ¼ cup shredded
cheddar cheese, ½ cup
fresh spinach, ½ cup fresh
tomatoes, 2 large tortillas

20 oz. water

## EVENING SNACK

1 macadamia-nut cookie with
white chocolate chips

# ALEX KOSTICH

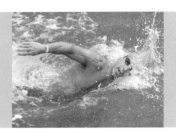

Alex Kostich is a highly decorated OPEN-WATER SWIMMER whose résumé includes three wins at the Waikiki Roughwater Swim and six wins at the La Jolla Rough Water Swim. Kostich, who was 42 years old when he logged the following food journal, also holds several age-group national records in the pool. The schedule of meals and workouts you see here is typical of his off-season, when Kostich swims less, lifts weights more, and eats less carbohydrate and more protein than he does during the racing season.

**WORKOUT 1** *(90 min. weight lifting)*
Water

**BREAKFAST**
20 oz. Isopure black tea

Banana

Chicken breast with Dijon mustard

**MORNING SNACK**
CLIF bar

16 oz. water

**WORKOUT 2** *(4-km swim)*
Water

**LUNCH**
6 oz. roast beef

Caesar salad with light dressing,
8 cherry tomatoes

½ cup black beans

½ cup butternut squash (boiled)

¼ fried plantain

16 oz. water

1 red velvet cupcake with
cream cheese frosting

**AFTERNOON SNACK**
1.75-oz. bag Chex Mix

**DINNER**
Sushi: spider roll, snow crab hand
roll, 2 pieces salmon, 2 pieces
salmon eggs, 2 pieces sweet
shrimp (and deep-fried heads),
lobster roll

# CHRISSIE WELLINGTON

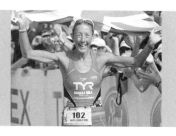

Chrissie Wellington of England is a TRIATHLETE who is a four-time winner of the Hawaii Ironman World Championship and holds the Ironman world record (8:33:56, set at Ironman South Africa in 2011). She notes that, in addition to the foods and drinks listed below, in a typical day she drinks water and Cytomax throughout the day (approximately 3 liters total).

**PREWORKOUT**
Banana with 2 Tbsp. honey,
2 Tbsp. peanut butter

Coffee with milk

**WORKOUT 1** *(swim)*

**BREAKFAST**
"Huge bowl" porridge oats,
all-bran buds, raisins, dried plums,
coconut, nuts, and seeds, mixed
with vanilla yogurt

Tea or coffee

**PREWORKOUT**
1 apple

**WORKOUT 2** *(ride)*
Cytomax sports drink

Muesli bar

Carbohydrate gel

**LUNCH**
2 bagel sandwiches with
turkey and cheese

Large green salad

Handful of nuts

**PREWORKOUT**
1 banana

**WORKOUT 3** *(run)*

**DINNER**
Beefsteak stir-fried with vegetables

Rice

Bowl of frozen fruit with yogurt

**EVENING SNACK**
1 small chocolate bar

# JOE DOMBROWSKI

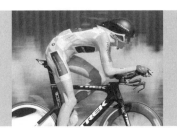

Joe Dombrowski is a **CYCLIST** who is one of America's most exciting young talents. A climbing specialist, "Dombro" had a breakout year in 2012, in which, at age 21, he finished 12th in the Tour of California and 3rd in the Tour of the Gila before winning the Girobio, known as the "Baby Giro d'Italia." The following food journal was recorded on a very hot training day at home in Marshall, Virginia, during which the young Team Sky member "drank water all day long" to stay hydrated.

**BREAKFAST**

2 slices whole wheat toast, 1 with peanut butter, 1 with raspberry jam

1 slice watermelon

Greek yogurt with granola and mixed nuts

Juice of 1 beet and 1 apple

Double espresso

**WORKOUT** *(3 hr. ride)*

4 bottles water with Base electrolyte salts

Banana

Honey Stinger bar

Peanut butter sandwich with maple syrup

**LUNCH**

Prosciutto sandwich made with whole wheat bread, asiago cheese, onion, arugula, pesto

Handful of tortilla chips with salsa

Fruit salad

Water

**AFTERNOON SNACK**

Plain frozen yogurt with blueberries and strawberries

**DINNER**

Beef burrito

Mixed green salad with olive oil and balsamic vinegar

1 slice watermelon, handful of strawberries

**EVENING SNACK**

Puffins cereal with milk

# SHALANE FLANAGAN

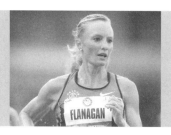

Shalane Flanagan is one of the most accomplished American RUNNERS in history. She has earned bronze medals in the 2008 Olympic 10,000 meters and the 2011 World Cross Country Championships. She holds American records for 10,000 meters (30:22.22), 5,000 meters indoors (14:47.32), and 3,000 meters indoors (8:33.25), and she previously held the record for 5,000 meters outdoors. Winner of 17 national championships in high school, college, and the professional ranks, Flanagan is also a three-time Olympic Trials winner. Here is an example of how Flanagan ate while preparing for the 2012 Olympic Marathon in London.

**BREAKFAST**
Oatmeal with honey, berries, banana slices, walnuts

Coffee with creamer

**WORKOUT 1** *(run plus gym session)*
Gatorade Endurance Formula

**LUNCH**
Large spinach salad with chicken, avocado, cheese, nuts, dried fruit

Yogurt

Whole wheat crackers

**WORKOUT 2** *(run)*
Gatorade Endurance Formula

**DINNER**
Steak

Steamed broccoli

Homemade sweet potato fries

**EVENING SNACK**
Dark chocolate

# ERIN CAFARO

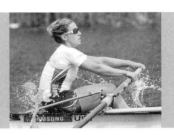

Erin Cafaro is a champion **ROWER** with an impressive collection of medals. She started with a bronze medal in the Women's 4- at the 2005 FISA U23 World Rowing Championships. She has since won three senior world championships gold medals and one bronze. In 2008 Cafaro was part of a team that won the first Olympic gold medal for the U.S. in the women's 8+. Four years later she successfully defended her Olympic title in London. Since 2009 Cafaro has followed the Paleo Diet, although she admits to retaining a tortilla chips vice.

**BREAKFAST 1**

Smoothie made with ½ cup frozen spinach, ½ frozen banana, ¼ cup frozen mango, 1 cup coconut milk, 1 scoop egg white protein, 2 scoops 3Fuel, and 1 Tbsp. Super Greens powder

**WORKOUT 1** *(rowing)*

**BREAKFAST 2**

3 eggs fried in grapeseed oil

2 cups kale with 2 Tbsp. olive oil, salt, pepper, lemon juice

3 pieces bacon

**LUNCH**

2 cups kale with 2 Tbsp. olive oil, salt, pepper, lemon juice, Dijon mustard

½ roasted chicken

¼ cup pistachios

5 strawberries

½ cup Trader Joe's roasted plantains

**PREWORKOUT**

2 scoops 3Fuel

**WORKOUT 2** *(weight lifting)*

**POSTWORKOUT**

1 apple

¼ cup peanut butter

**DINNER**

Burger made with ¼ lb. grass-fed beef, ¼ lb. bison, 2 pieces bacon

½ cup sautéed mushrooms

¼ cup sautéed onions

1½ cups Brussels sprout salad made with shredded Brussels sprouts, roasted hazelnuts, salt, pepper, lemon juice, olive oil, Dijon mustard

**EVENING SNACK**

1 pear

# SCOTT JUREK

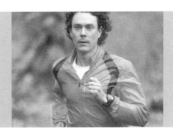

Scott Jurek of Seattle, Washington, is one of America's most accomplished ULTRARUNNERS. He has won the Western States 100 seven times, the Badwater Ultramarathon twice, and many other major ultramarathons around the world. He is also a vegan, which means he consumes no animal or animal-derived foods of any kind. Jurek explains his diet: "I eat organic foods as much as possible (probably 90 percent of my diet), and I have been trying to eat more locally grown, seasonal foods. I try to get people to think about what I eat rather than what I do not eat, as that is how I look at it." As a vegan, Jurek recognizes the importance of finding healthy alternatives when he chooses to cut something out of his diet. He focuses on eating healthy fats, whole grains, legumes, soy protein (via tempeh, tofu, miso, and fermented soy powder), nuts, seeds, fruits, and vegetables. During peak training Jurek eats about 5,000 calories a day. Here's a one-day snapshot of his diet.

**WORKOUT 1**
*(run, core strength, stretching)*
CLIF shot electrolyte drink

Water

**BREAKFAST**
2–3 servings Green Magma probiotics supplement

Carbohydrate-protein smoothie (usually a mix of soaked almonds, dates, hempseeds, bananas, blueberries, hemp protein and/ or fermented soy protein powder, vanilla, maca powder, sea salt)

1–2 servings soy yogurt mixed with 2–3 Tbsp. ground flaxseeds

3–4 pieces whole fruit

2–4 cups whole-grain cereal with dried fruit (muesli or hot cereal, mixed-grain porridge or polenta, or raw buckwheat porridge)

2–4 slices Ezekiel sprouted-grain bread with 2–4 Tbsp. raw almond butter

**MORNING SNACK**

Herbal tea (raw yerba maté or green tea) or, rarely, one shot of espresso

Fruit or energy bar

**LUNCH**

Large mixed green salad made with dark leafy greens, sprouts, raw kale, arugula, etc., with tomatoes, cucumbers, carrots, etc.

Whole grains or whole-grain pasta or bread

Legumes (beans or lentils)

**AFTERNOON SNACK**

Fruit, energy bar, nuts, seeds, or dried fruit

**WORKOUT 2** *(run)*

CLIF shot electrolyte drink
Water

**DINNER**

Large salad (similar to lunch but with different greens and veggies, such as raw cabbage) or steamed/ sautéed dark greens (such as kale or collards), steamed vegetables, sautéed tofu, tempeh, or legumes (lentils, pinto beans, or garbanzo beans)

Potatoes, yams, squash, or whole-grain/sprouted pasta or whole grains (brown rice, quinoa, etc.)

**EVENING SNACK**

Homemade mixture of fresh fruit, dates, nuts or dark chocolate

# SARAH HASKINS

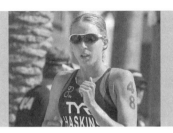

Sarah Haskins is a top American **SHORT-COURSE TRIATHLETE**. Her résumé includes a silver medal at the 2008 ITU Triathlon World Championships, a victory at the 2011 Pan-American Games, and an 11th-place finish at the 2012 Olympics in Beijing. Especially dominant in non-drafting triathlons, Haskins has won St. Anthony's Triathlon, the Chicago Triathlon, the Los Angeles Triathlon, and more than 20 others. Here's what she ate and drank during a training day at the end of the 2012 season.

**BREAKFAST 1**
1 slice whole wheat toast with
1 sliced banana, 2 Tbsp. natural
peanut butter, honey

Water

Cup hot natural cocoa

**WORKOUT 1** *(10-mile run)*
20 oz. PowerBar Perform drink

**BREAKFAST 2**
12 oz. smoothie made with
carrot juice, beet juice, blueberries,
almond milk, ½ banana, ice

Water

1 apple

**LUNCH**
1 cup Greek yogurt with honey,
banana, almonds

**WORKOUT 2** *(5,000-m swim)*
20 oz. PowerBar Perform drink

**POSTWORKOUT**
1 apple

1 Tbsp. natural peanut butter
with celery

Water

½ cup cherry juice

**WORKOUT 3** *(60 min. easy spin on bike)*
20 oz. water

**DINNER**
6 oz. ham

Salad made with spinach,
tomato, broccoli, feta cheese,
balsamic vinaigrette dressing

Water

**EVENING SNACK**
1 cup popcorn popped with
coconut oil

1 cup almond milk

# DOTSIE BAUSCH

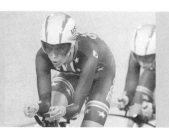

Dotsie Bausch is a TRACK CYCLIST whose career highlights include seven national championship titles and two Pan-Am Games gold medals. In 2012 Bausch won a silver medal for the U.S. in the team pursuit at the London Olympics. A former fashion model, Bausch took up cycling at age 26 as part of her recovery from anorexia and cocaine addiction. (Note: Dotsie drinks coffee right after she wakes up.)

**BREAKFAST**

3 scrambled egg whites with spring onions and sliced tomatoes

1 slice dark whole-grain German bread with Smart Balance and ½ avocado

**PREWORKOUT**

Smoothie made with 1 banana, 2 cups cold water and ice, 1 cup blueberries, 1 Tbsp. ground flaxseed, 1 Tbsp. hemp protein, 1 Tbsp. agave nectar, 1 Tbsp. hemp oil, 2 tsp. ground rooibos, 3–4 dashes cinnamon

**WORKOUT** (ride)

Bonk Breaker Bar

**LUNCH**

Large salad "with a variety of whatever is in the house" (e.g., spinach, garbanzo beans, kidney beans, tomatoes, flaxseeds, carrots, pomegranate seeds, celery, slivered almonds, mushrooms) dressed with rice vinegar and a homemade blend of pumpkin-seed oil, flaxseed oil, hempseed oil, salt, and pepper

**DINNER**

Steamed kale with lemon, diced peppers, and oil and vinegar

Whole-grain pasta or rice or potatoes

Large salad similar to lunch

Toasted bread with pesto and fresh roasted garlic cloves

1 glass red wine

**EVENING SNACK**

1–2 squares dark chocolate and frozen blueberries

# HUNTER KEMPER

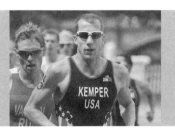

Hunter Kemper is a four-time U.S. Olympian in **TRIATHLON**, a seven-time national champion, and a two-time Pan Am Games medalist. Here's what Kemper eats on a typical training day.

**BREAKFAST 1**

Wheaties with flaxseed sprinkled on top, skim milk

**PREWORKOUT**

1 banana

**WORKOUT 1** *(swim)*

24 oz. Amino Vital Endurance

**POSTWORKOUT**

Protein bar with at least 20 g protein

**WORKOUT 2** *(run)*

16 oz. Amino Vital Endurance

**BREAKFAST 2**

3- or 4-egg omelet with vegetables, ham, American cheese

Plain bagel

2 small pancakes, lightly buttered

16 oz. fruit smoothie with a spoonful of flaxseed

16 oz. Amino Vital Pro

8 oz. orange juice

**LUNCH**

Turkey and cheese sandwich
on a toasted whole wheat bagel

24 oz. Amino Vital Pro

1 cup strawberry-banana yogurt

16 oz. water

Fruit medley (sliced apple, sliced
banana, grapes, strawberries)

**WORKOUT 3** *(ride)*

48 oz. Amino Vital Endurance

1 carbohydrate gel

1 energy bar

**POSTWORKOUT**

Protein bar with at least
20 g protein

24 oz. water

24 oz. Amino Vital Pro for
afternoon hydration

**DINNER**

Salad with feta cheese,
pecans, sesame dressing

Full plate pasta with
grilled chicken breast

2 slices garlic toast

24 oz. water

**EVENING SNACK**

Wheaties with skim milk and raisins

# GEORGIA GOULD

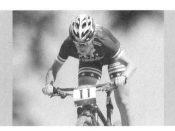

Georgia Gould is a five-time U.S. national champion in **MOUNTAIN BIKING** who competes for the LUNA Chix Pro Team. In the winter Gould trades her fat tires for a cyclocross bike, on which she also excels, winning the U.S. Gran Prix of Cyclocross Series three times. The following food journal was recorded just a few weeks before Gould won the bronze medal in the 2012 Olympic Cross Country Mountain Bike event.

**BREAKFAST**

Cornflakes and granola with plain yogurt, blueberries, banana

1 French press yerba maté tea

**MORNING SNACK**

Couple of handfuls trail mix

20 oz. ginger tea

**LUNCH**

2 fried eggs over arugula, artichoke hearts, olives, cherry tomatoes

A few gluten-free crackers

**WORKOUT** *(1 hr. recovery ride)*

1 bottle water

**DINNER**

Grass-fed steak

Roasted beets and rutabaga

Sautéed zucchini with onions and basil

Watercress salad with artichoke hearts, olives, feta cheese, tomatoes, olive oil, balsamic vinegar

20 oz. herbal tea

# SHANNON ROWBURY

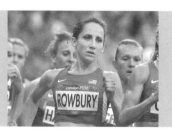

Shannon Rowbury of San Francisco, California, is a MIDDLE-DISTANCE RUNNER whose achievements include an NCAA national championship title in the mile and U.S. national championship titles at 1,500, 3,000 meters, and the road mile. She represented the United States in the 1,500 m at both the 2008 and the 2012 Olympics, earning a spot in the final in Beijing.

**BREAKFAST**
½ sprouted-grain English muffin with local honey, chunky almond butter

½ banana

Dark-roast coffee with lots of milk

Water

**WORKOUT 1** *(run)*
Carbohydrate-protein sports drink

**POSTWORKOUT**
½ protein bar

1 apple

Water

**LUNCH**
2 eggs scrambled with onion, mushroom, spinach, vine-ripened tomato, sundried tomato, tofu, mozzarella

Water

**WORKOUT 2** *(run)*
Carbohydrate-protein sports drink

**AFTERNOON SNACK**
Carrots

Water

**DINNER**
Broiled salmon

Quinoa

Salad made with romaine lettuce, avocado, carrots, tomatoes, olive oil, balsamic vinegar

Water

1 piece dark chocolate

**EVENING SNACK**
Protein powder with milk

# LUCAS VERZBICAS

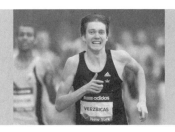

Lucas Verzbicas was only 19 years old at the time of this writing but had already amassed a career's worth of achievements as a **TRIATHLETE** and **RUNNER**. As a high school student in Orland Park, Illinois, he won the Foot Locker High School Cross Country Championship twice, set a national high school 2-mile record of 8:29, and became only the fifth American high school student to break 4 minutes for the mile. He won the Duathlon World Junior Championships in 2009 and the ITU Triathlon World Junior Championships in 2011. Verzbicas was a resident athlete at the U.S. Olympic Training Center in Colorado Springs and eating most of his meals at the center's cafeteria when he recorded the following food journal.

**PREWORKOUT**
2 scoops Herbalife 24
Formula 1 Sport

**WORKOUT 1** *(swim plus run)*
Water

**BREAKFAST**
3 Tbsp. Greek yogurt with
2 sliced grapefruits

3-egg omelet with spinach, sliced
tomatoes, shredded pepper jack
cheese, sliced green peppers

Iced green tea

**LUNCH**
Mixed steamed vegetables

Mixed bean salad

2 Tbsp. chia seeds soaked in water

Iron supplement

**WORKOUT 2** *(run)*
Herbalife 24 Hydrate

**POSTWORKOUT**
Herbalife 24 Rebuild Endurance

**DINNER**
Beef stroganoff with noodles,
roasted asparagus

Spinach salad with tomatoes,
cabbage, carrots, red pepper

Multivitamin

**EVENING SNACK**
McDonald's soft-serve
frozen yogurt

Herbalife 24 Restore

# SHELLEY OLDS

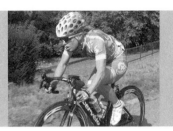

Shelley Olds is a world-class **TRACK AND ROAD CYCLIST**. She has twice won the U.S. National Track Championships gold medal. Her major road victories include the 2010 Pan-American Games Road Race, the 2010 U.S. National Criterium Championships, and the 2010 Tour of New Zealand. She finished 7th in the 2012 Olympic Road Race. Following is Olds's diet on an average training day.

**BREAKFAST**

2 cups cereal with milk and bananas

Coffee with milk

**WORKOUT** *(3 to 4 hr. ride)*

Water

Water with electrolytes

1 banana

**LUNCH**

2 fillets chicken with onion and apple

1 cup white rice

1 cup peas

Water with lemon

**DINNER**

Large salad with olives, tomatoes, peppers, onion, carrots, balsamic vinegar

2 fillets salmon

Water with lemon

# MAX KING

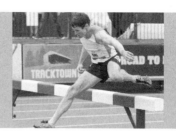

Max King is one of the most versatile American **RUNNERS**. He has excelled on the track (finishing 5th in the 2005 USA Outdoor Track and Field Championships steeplechase), as a cross-country runner (representing the U.S. in multiple World Cross Country Championships), on the roads (he has a 29:01 road 10K PR), and as a trail runner (winning four consecutive XTERRA Trail Run World Championship titles). Recently his focus has turned to ultramarathons, where he's had even greater success, winning the 2011 U.S. 50K Trail Championship.

**BREAKFAST**

Cup of granola with 8 oz. 2% milk

3 small eggs

**WORKOUT 1** *(90 min. easy mountain run)*

**POSTWORKOUT**

2 pieces of toast (whole wheat with seeds) with 2 Tbsp. Udo's Omega 3, 6, 9 Oil

16 oz. smoothie made with yogurt, ice cream, blueberries, green foods powder, strawberries, mango, banana

**LUNCH**

Peanut butter and jelly sandwich with 1 Tbsp. peanut butter and 1 Tbsp. jelly

Large chocolate chip cookie

Hammer Bar

**WORKOUT 2** *(50 min. easy run)*

**DINNER**

3 cups chickpea soup made with chickpeas, kale, tomatoes, garlic, broth

2 Tbsp. elderberry extract

6 oz. milk

**EVENING SNACK**

14 oz. smoothie

1 cup mint chocolate chip ice cream

## YOUR RACING WEIGHT DIET

Few, if any, of the athletes whose eating habits we've glimpsed in this chapter follow the same diet today that they followed before they became world-class athletes. Most young endurance athletes with world-class talent change their eating habits to some degree to aid their performance by attaining racing weight and other means. In almost every case this process entails an elevation of diet quality, but each athlete finds his or her own way to do so. Many factors, including personal tastes, nutrition and food knowledge, and cooking skills, influence the individual paths of diet evolution that great athletes find. Similar influences will shape the development of your Racing Weight diet. As long as you stay within the parameters of the system, there is no wrong path.

# THIRTEEN

# RACING WEIGHT AND YOU

I receive a lot of questions about the Racing Weight system from athletes of all kinds. A majority of the questions come from members of special populations within the endurance sports community who want to know how to make the Racing Weight system work best for them. While the program is truly for everyone, individual athletes must practice it in slightly different ways. For example, a vegan runner and her gluten-free husband can both follow all six steps of the Racing Weight system, but they will probably eat many different foods.

There are six special populations of the endurance sports community that I hear from most often: athletes with past or present eating disorders, athletes seeking to lose muscle weight, gluten-free athletes, vegetarians and vegans, older athletes, and young athletes. This chapter will offer special guidelines for each of these six groups.

## ATHLETES WITH PAST OR PRESENT EATING DISORDERS AND BODY DYSMORPHIA

Some nonathletes think that every lean endurance athlete who complains about not being lean enough must have an eating disorder or body dysmorphia (self-obsession with perceived flaw's in a person's body). In fact, most endurance athletes who are dissatisfied with their current weight are healthy eaters with a realistic body image. We complain about our bodies because we know that if we were a bit leaner, we would race a litter faster (and, yes, maybe look even better).

Research suggests that endurance athletes generally have a slightly more favorable body image than nonathletes. This is what we would expect to see if athletes and nonathletes were completely objective about their bodies, because, owing to their training, endurance athletes typically have bodies that look more like the social ideal. A West Chester University study involving 62 female college swimmers reported that the average score on the standard Social Physique Anxiety Scale (SPAS) fell in the "low healthy" range (Reel 1997). The authors of the study noted that a sizable portion of the body anxiety these women did feel came from their wearing revealing swimsuits in a group environment for two or more hours a day every day. If nonathletes had to do the same, their SPAS score would probably increase substantially!

## ATHLETES FACE GREAT PRESSURE TO BE THIN BECAUSE OF THE CONNECTION BETWEEN LEANNESS AND PERFORMANCE.

Some of the swimmers in this study did have an unhealthy body image, however, as does a minority of athletes of both genders in all endurance sports. A negative body image is not only a source of unhappiness but is also often the cause of disordered eating. Female runners in high school and college are especially prone to developing eating disorders. The pressure to be thin puts all young women at risk of becoming anorexic or bulimic, but athletes face even greater pressure because of the connection between leanness and performance. Forty-two percent of the swimmers included in the West Chester study believed that they would perform better if they lost weight. Most of these women were probably right—they would have performed better if they had lost a little excess body fat *the right way*. But what seems to happen too often with young female athletes especially is that the desire to lose weight for performance gets mixed up with the desire to lose weight to look like a catalog model, and weight loss is then sought the wrong way—through undereating, purging, and/or overtraining.

The terrible irony is that disordered eating never improves performance in the long term, and it never improves anyone's appearance either. So endurance athletes have no rational reason to maintain an eating disorder, but unfortunately eating disorders are a form of mental illness that are not affected by rational calculations. I have a friend who wrote a school report about anorexia in middle school and became anorexic in high school. Her knowledge of the subject could not protect her.

I am not qualified to counsel athletes with past or present body dysmorphia disorders or eating disorders, and I never try to. Nor, thankfully, am I often asked to. What athletes who have dealt with or are dealing with such issues do ask me sometimes is whether it is "okay" for them to follow the Racing Weight system. All I can say is that I have every confidence that this system represents the right way—the healthy way—to manage weight as an endurance athlete. If you follow the six steps in the proper spirit, your eating will not be disordered and you will not become unhealthy. But it is possible to pursue the program in the wrong spirit, with an unhealthy obsession to become unrealistically skinny, and if there is even the remotest chance of this happening with you, then you should skip the program and seek qualified counseling instead.

When this book was first published, an interviewer from a running Web site stunned me by asking if I feared that I would be accused of encouraging eating disorders by openly advocating performance weight management. The idea had never crossed my mind. I've had a few years to think about this question, and I feel no less certain that this book is part of the solution, not a contributor to the problem. Too often athletes pursue weight loss in secret and the wrong way. I feel that *Racing Weight* has brought performance weight management out into the open where it should be and shown athletes the right way to tackle it. Now we must all work together to change the environment that causes so many athletes to try to get as skinny as possible at all costs.

## ATHLETES SEEKING TO LOSE MUSCLE WEIGHT

Excess muscle weight is not quite as detrimental to endurance performance as excess body fat, but it is detrimental. That's why you are no more likely to see a muscle-bound person at the front of a race than an obese person. Losing excess muscle the right way therefore does improve endurance performance.

It is not possible to predict how much muscle mass is expendable. If you lose too much, your performance will suffer. So it's best not to set a goal for muscle mass loss and just focus on losing it the right way.

The right way to lose excess muscle mass has been demonstrated by successful endurance athletes who were heavily muscled when they started their sport. One such person is Troy Jacobson, a top professional triathlete of the 1990s who played football before that. "I weighed in at 220 pounds in my senior year in high school and spent all my time in the weight room and drank a gallon of milk a day in order to continue to gain weight," Jacobson once told me in an interview for *Triathlete*. "I was captain of the football team, captain of the wrestling team, and a heavyweight wrestler. I was one of the guys who would make fun of the skinny dudes running around the track."

## HIGH-VOLUME, LOW-INTENSITY TRAINING IS THE MOST EFFECTIVE METHOD OF LOSING EXCESS MUSCLE MASS.

Upon quitting football and training for his first triathlon in college, Jacobson quickly lost 30 pounds of excess muscle mass. He would lose almost another 30 before it was all said and done. The key to his success in attaining a racing weight that enabled him to win such major triathlons as Blackwater Eagleman and the Buffalo Springs Lake Triathlon was a high-volume training program that included plenty of low-intensity workouts to ensure that the volume was manageable.

Other cases similar to Jacobson's confirm that high-volume, low-intensity training is the most effective method of losing excess muscle mass. This type of training causes individual muscle fibers to become thinner, so the muscles as a whole effectively deflate and the athlete loses weight even though the total number of muscle fibers doesn't change. High-volume, low-intensity running is especially effective. Even if you're a cyclist or a swimmer, you may want to incorporate running into your training if you have excess muscle mass to lose. Troy Jacobson ran marathons outside of triathlon season as a way to get skinnier, setting an impressive personal best of 2:31:40 three weeks after the 1993 Ironman World Championship.

You should also avoid heavy weight lifting if you're trying to shed muscle weight. Limit your strength training to body-weight exercises for the core, hips, and other muscles that may need to be strengthened to improve joint stability and avoid injury. In other words, avoid exercises such as the Barbell Squat (page 247) and focus on exercises like the X-Band Walk (page 252). Yoga is okay too because it strengthens the muscles without building them up.

As for diet, there are two effective ways to eat for muscle loss. The fastest way is to maintain a large energy deficit, but the best way is to follow the Racing Weight diet steps. A lot of energy is required to maintain muscle mass, and when the diet does not provide sufficient energy, some muscle proteins are broken down to supply energy to other muscle cells. Known as catabolism, or "muscle cannibalism," this process is harmful to endurance performance. To lose muscle without hurting your performance, simply follow the four dietary steps of the Racing Weight system: improve your diet quality, balance your energy sources, manage your appetite, and time your meals and snacks appropriately.

# GLUTEN-FREE ATHLETES

Gluten is a protein in wheat and a few other grains that has damaging effects in approximately 0.7 percent of the population (Rubio-Tapia et al. 2012). Persons with Celiac disease have a genetic predisposition that does not allow them to safely consume any gluten. Others are merely gluten-intolerant, lacking the genetic predisposition but suffering similar symptoms (which range from diarrhea to skin rashes) after eating gluten-containing foods. Still others are gluten-sensitive: They don't feel great after consuming gluten but they can consume it in small amounts without any real harm.

Gluten-free diets have become extremely popular in recent years. Most of the people on them do not need to be. The alarm that has been stoked around Celiac disease, gluten intolerance, and gluten sensitivity has given many the idea that gluten is a poison that nobody should eat. Nothing could be further from the truth. Gluten is not only harmless but also nourishing to the vast majority of people.

"Someone who needs to be on a gluten-free diet and is closely monitored can benefit tremendously from it," said Dr. Stefano Guandalini, medical director at the University of Chicago Celiac Disease Center, in a 2012 interview for WebMD. "But for everyone else, embracing this diet makes no sense" (Boyles 2012).

While I look forward to the day when wheat and other grains are no longer unfairly vilified, in the meantime I see no real harm in the gluten-free diet phenomenon. Athletes who have gone gluten free either by necessity or by choice often ask me whether it is compatible with the Racing Weight system. Most sensible diets are compatible with the Racing Weight system, and gluten-free diets are no exception.

Gluten is found in most breads and other baked goods, pastas, breakfast cereals, crackers, and beers, as well as in a host of other random things such as soy sauce. When you eliminate all of these foods from your diet, there are still plenty of others left to eat—all fruits and vegetables, all seeds and nuts, all lean meats and fish, and even some grain-based foods, including those made with rice, corn, and oats.

The typical American gets a sizable percentage of daily carbohydrates from foods that contain gluten. Many endurance athletes do too. These athletes also often do not consume enough carbs, and the removal of wheat, barley, and rye from the diet might increase their shortfall if they're not careful. My one word of caution for gluten-free endurance athletes is this: Be extra vigilant in your efforts to meet your body's carbohydrate needs.

## VEGETARIANS AND VEGANS

Americans eat more meat than anyone else in the world, but lately we've begun to eat less. Between 2007 and 2012 meat consumption decreased by more than 12 percent. While economic factors are partly responsible for the decline, its main cause appears to be health concerns. Meat is viewed increasingly as unhealthy, or at least less healthy than other foods.

There are numbers that back up this belief. In Chapter 4 I mentioned a study that found that regular meat consumption was associated with almost a pound of weight gain every four years, whereas fruits, vegetables, and some other foods attenuated long-term weight gain.

Some experts maintain that any amount of meat in the diet is unhealthy. One such expert is Colin Campbell, a Cornell University nutritionist who authored *The China Study* and was featured in the documentary film *Forks over Knives*. In an interview for the *New York Times*, Campbell stated, "I say the closer we get to a plant-based diet the healthier we are going to be" (Parker-Pope 2011).

Most experts disagree with this position. I certainly do. Campbell relies too heavily on epidemiological data and not enough on common sense to support his thesis. It's true that heavy meat eaters are more likely to develop some cancers and heart disease than those who eat little or no meat, but this doesn't lead to the conclusion that meat in general is unhealthy. The few studies that have looked at the health effects of particular kinds of meat have generally found that certain meats are perfectly healthy. For example, a comprehensive review of 1,600 past studies conducted by researchers at the Harvard School of Public Health found that only processed meats (such as hot dogs, sausage, and many cold cuts) were associated with increased risk for cardiovascular disease and diabetes, whereas unprocessed meats were not (Micha, Wallace, and Mozzafarian 2010).

The typical meat lover does not limit his animal-food intake to lean cuts of grass-fed beef and fresh fish, or complement his meat eating with a heavy intake of fresh fruits and vegetables, or exercise vigorously every day. It's unreasonable to suggest that atypical meat eaters who do these things are jeopardizing their health in a way that vegans are not. It would be nice to have a study that confirms my viewpoint, but in the meantime it's undeniable that the vast majority of the world's best endurance athletes—who are among the world's healthiest humans—eat meat.

As I stated in Chapter 3, I am not in favor of artificial dietary restrictions or forbidden foods. If you want to avoid all sweets or all fried foods, go ahead. But I think it's best to eat all six of the high-quality food categories: vegetables, fruits, nuts and seeds, lean meats and fish, whole grains, and dairy. Each is good in a slightly different way from the others, so why not include all of them in your diet?

This is not to say that a person cannot achieve optimal health, or that an athlete cannot achieve optimal performance, on a diet that excludes one or more of the high-quality food groups. Only vegetables and fruits are essential to optimal health and performance. You can thrive on these foods alone. Vegetarians eat only vegetables, fruits, nuts and seeds, whole grains, and dairy foods among the six categories of high-quality foods. Vegans eat only the first four. There are many successful vegetarian and vegan endurance athletes.

TABLE 13.1 **HOW TO SCORE VEGETARIAN OR VEGAN DIETS**

|  | FOOD TYPE | SERVING NUMBER | | | | | |
|---|---|---|---|---|---|---|---|
|  |  | 1ST | 2ND | 3RD | 4TH | 5TH | 6TH |
| **HIGH** QUALITY | Fruits | 2 | 2 | 2 | 1 | 0 | 0 |
|  | Vegetables | 2 | 2 | 2 | 1 | 0 | 0 |
|  | Legumes & plant proteins | 2 | 2 | 1 | 0 | 0 | -1 |
|  | Nuts & seeds | 2 | 2 | 1 | 0 | 0 | -1 |
|  | Whole grains | 2 | 2 | 1 | 0 | 0 | -1 |
|  | Dairy | 1 | 1 | 1 | 0 | -1 | -2 |
| **LOW** QUALITY | Refined grains | -1 | -1 | -2 | -2 | -2 | -2 |
|  | Sweets | -2 | -2 | -2 | -2 | -2 | -2 |
|  | Fried foods | -2 | -2 | -2 | -2 | -2 | -2 |
|  | Fatty proteins | -1 | -1 | -2 | -2 | -2 | -2 |

The question I receive most often from such athletes concerns how to use the Diet Quality Score on a vegetarian or vegan diet. It can be as simple as adjusting the maximum score from 32 for omnivores to 27 for vegetarians and 24 for vegans. Another option is to replace the lean meats and fish category with a new category of high-protein plant foods (Table 13.1). This category includes legumes (which are no longer counted as vegetables), hemp seeds, spirulina, high-protein plant-based packaged foods and supplements, and all other plant-based foods besides nuts and seeds that provide more than 5 grams of protein per serving.

Getting enough protein is generally considered to be the greatest nutritional challenge for vegetarians and vegans, but this concern is overblown. Humans don't need a lot of protein—10 percent of total calories will do the job—and plant foods are more than adequate to meet that need. Vegetarians and especially vegans are more likely to fall short of meeting their needs for vitamin B12, vitamin D, calcium, and iron.

To avoid a deficiency in vitamins B12 and D, take a daily multivitamin supplement that contains both. To avoid a calcium deficiency, eat plenty of calcium-rich plant foods, such as kale, spinach, sesame seeds, and broccoli. To prevent an iron deficiency, eat plenty of whole grains and legumes and have your iron level checked by a physician once a year.

# OLDER ATHLETES

Alex Kostich, whom we first met in Chapter 12, is one of the most decorated open-water swimmers in history. He has won the La Jolla Roughwater swim six times, the Waikiki Roughwater Swim three times, and countless other major events. Now in his 40s, Kostich continues to compete at the highest level of the sport. But it's not because his body is impervious to the effects of aging.

Kostich noticed the first bodily sign of aging right around the time he turned 30. "Almost overnight I noticed that I started gaining weight if I wasn't careful with my diet," he says. Determined to stay lean and keep winning, Kostich became more austere in his eating habits. (See Kostich's one-day food journal on page 210.) He also added running to his training regimen to burn off extra fat, and he increased his commitment to weight lifting to maintain his lean muscle mass.

Many endurance athletes discover that weight management becomes more difficult as they get older. It is not entirely clear why this happens. While weight gain in aging nonathletes is associated with declining muscle mass and a concomitant drop in metabolism, research has shown that athletes are able to preserve their muscle mass and metabolic rate through training. It's possible that changes in hormones, including decreased estrogen production in women and declining testosterone production in men, are at least partly responsible for the greater difficulty of racing weight maintenance that older athletes often experience. Whatever the cause, the phenomenon is normal and indeed almost universal.

If and when you notice that it's getting harder to attain or maintain your racing weight, respond by stepping up your commitment to the Racing Weight system. There is some room for improvement in every athlete's weight-management practices. Once you've been at it for a while, you will have a clear understanding of where the slack is in your execution of the system. Perhaps your average DQS could be a little higher or you could get a little more serious about managing your appetite. Identify one or two ways to step up your weight-management efforts and execute them. Chances are they will counteract the aging processes that are making you more prone to weight gain.

Don't expect to stop the clock, however. Even athletes who are very dedicated to weight management often find that they cannot race at the same weight or body-fat percentage after age 40 or 50 as they did when they were younger. One of the reasons is that body fat slowly accumulates around the visceral organs throughout adulthood. Whereas fat accumulation close to the surface of the body can be prevented through diet and training, visceral fat accumulation cannot. Don't frustrate yourself by refusing to adjust your racing weight to account for age. Don't give up, either. Just continue to practice the Racing Weight system; monitor your weight, body-fat percentage, and performance; and make a sensible change.

# YOUNG ATHLETES

How young is too young to start thinking about racing weight? This is a question I hear sometimes from the mothers and fathers of teenage endurance athletes. These parents express a concern that their children might develop an unhealthy preoccupation with their weight at an age when the risk for such anxieties is especially high.

This is a legitimate concern, but my own greatest concern about the pursuit of racing weight in high school athletes is different. Most athletes of this age are still growing, "filling out," and going through puberty. This reality makes the individual's racing weight a moving target—impossible to determine and therefore pointless to pursue as adult athletes do.

As a high school sophomore in Minneapolis, Kara Goucher (then Kara Wheeler) qualified for the Foot Locker High School Cross Country Championship. She was barely 5 feet tall and weighed less than 90 pounds. She finished 9th. When she returned to Foot Locker the next year, Goucher was 3 inches taller and 15 pounds heavier. She finished 16th. By the time she graduated from high school, Goucher was 5'5" and weighed 125 pounds. "I grew so fast, it hurt," she told me.

This is a normal pattern for female high school runners. Freshmen and sophomores dominate, but the best runners typically plateau or even slide backward in their last two years of high school because their chassis are growing faster than their engines, so to speak. If they stick with the sport, they start improving again in college after growth and puberty are behind them. Kara Goucher was terribly frustrated by her failure to keep improving in high school, and so are most runners who share this common experience. Trying to push past the performance plateau through performance weight management would only compound the frustration. Nature must take its course.

Young female athletes in other sports experience milder plateaus, and young male athletes in all endurance sports typically don't have them at all. But all these athletes are still growing, so it doesn't make any more sense for them to determine and pursue a specific racing weight.

## NO ENDURANCE ATHLETE IS TOO YOUNG TO EAT RIGHT, TRAIN SMART, OR LEARN.

I advise the parents of teenage endurance athletes to stay mum on the subject of weight unless their children bring it up. The last thing you want to do is be another source of pressure to be skinny. If your child expresses an interest in performance weight management, give her these very words to read, or summarize them for her. Make crystal clear to your young athlete that the numbers on the bathroom scale have no meaning yet.

No endurance athlete is too young to eat right, train smart, or learn, however. The next thing you should do for a child who shows an interest in performance weight management after giving her these words to read is to encourage her to read the rest of the book. If your child expresses a desire to practice the Racing Weight system, let her implement every step except for self-monitoring. Improving diet quality, balancing energy sources, managing appetite, practicing nutrient timing, and training properly will help your young athlete improve even if she doesn't use these steps to attain a specific racing weight.

If you have individual concerns about adapting the Racing Weight system to your needs that are not addressed here, please contact me through my Web site: mattfitzgerald.org.

# STRENGTH EXERCISES FOR ENDURANCE ATHLETES

The following are 30 strength exercises for endurance athletes: five each for all endurance athletes, cross-country skiers, cyclists, rowers, runners, swimmers, and triathletes. Note that the five strength exercises for triathletes draw one from the list for cyclists, two from the list for runners, and two from the list for swimmers.

It is wise to start with an adaptation phase if these exercises are new or you are not currently strength training. Spend two to three weeks practicing the movements with very light loads (in the case of non-bodyweight exercises) to get the coordination down. Then you can move on to heavier loads. As you might recall from Chapter 9, you want to work up to the heavier loads because they complement your endurance training, building power and a leaner body.

# EXERCISES FOR ALL ENDURANCE ATHLETES

## 1 SIDE PLANK
**Strengthens the lateral core stabilizers to improve the stability of the spine, pelvis, and hips during athletic activities**

Lie on your side with your ankles together and your torso propped up by your upper arm. Lift your hips upward until your body forms a diagonal plank from ankles to neck. Hold this position for 20 to 30 seconds, making sure you don't allow your hips to sag toward the floor. (Watch yourself in a mirror to make sure you're not sagging.) Switch to the other side, and repeat the exercise.

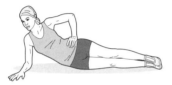 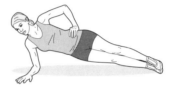

## 2 SUPINE PLANK
**Strengthens the gluteals and hamstrings**

Lie face up on the floor with your knees bent 90 degrees and your feet flat on the floor. Contract your gluteals and lift your hips until your body forms a straight line from neck to knees. Hold this position for 5 seconds, keeping your buttocks squeezed together; then return to the starting position. Complete 10 repetitions.

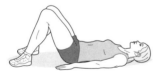 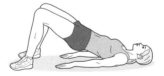

## 3 PRONE PLANK
### Builds the endurance of the spinal stabilizers

Lie on the floor on your stomach, with your upper body supported on your forearms and your toes pressed into the ground. Maintain a 90-degree bend in your elbows, and make sure they are placed directly underneath the shoulders. Tighten your entire core area, and lift your hips up and in line with your legs and torso. Hold this position for up to 30 seconds without allowing your hips to sag. If you can hold the prone plank position longer than 30 seconds, make it more challenging by doing it with your left foot elevated a few inches above the floor for 15 seconds, then your right foot elevated for 15 seconds.

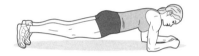 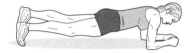

## 4 CABLE TRUNK ROTATION
### Strengthens the trunk rotational stabilizers to improve the stability of the spine, pelvis, and hips during athletic activities

Stand with your left side facing a cable pulley station. Attach a D-handle at shoulder height, and begin with your trunk rotated toward the weight stack and your arms fully extended with the handle grasped in both hands. Keeping your arms extended and your hands in line with the center of your chest, rotate your trunk 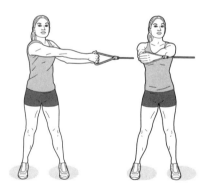 to the right. Keep your abdominal muscles tightened, and avoid hunching your shoulders as you do so. Stop when your hands are at about the "1 or 2 o'clock" position (with the "12 o'clock" position being hands directly out in front of you); then return to the starting position. Repeat 10 to 12 times; then reverse your position, and perform a set twisting in the opposite direction.

# 5 SWISS BALL HYPEREXTENSION
**Strengthens the lower back muscles to improve the stability of the spine, pelvis, and hips during athletic activities**

Lie face down on a Swiss ball with your upper thighs, pelvic area, and stomach supported by the ball and only your toes touching the floor and your arms extended directly forward, Superman-style. Contract your lower back muscles, and lift your torso upward, keeping your arms in line with your spine. Extend your spine as much as possible; then return to the starting position. Repeat 12 to 15 times.

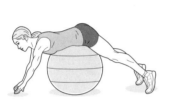

# STRENGTH EXERCISES FOR CROSS-COUNTRY SKIERS

# 1 ROMANIAN DEADLIFT
**Strengthens the hamstrings, gluteals, and lower back for more powerful leg action**

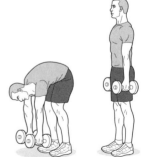

Stand with your feet close together, knees bent very slightly, with a dumbbell next to each foot. Set your core, and then bend forward at the waist and grab the dumbbells. With arms at your side and knees locked in the slightly bent position, return to a standing position. Pause briefly, and then bend forward to do another repetition. Complete 10 to 12 repetitions in total.

## 2 STEP-UP
**Strengthens the gluteals, hamstrings, and quadriceps and corrects muscular imbalance in the thigh muscles**

Stand facing an exercise bench or a step (12 to 18 inches high) while holding a dumbbell in each hand at your sides. Step up onto the bench with your right foot, and then push off your right heel as you raise your left leg so that you're standing on the bench. Step back down with your left leg. Continue stepping up and down, pushing with your right leg and carrying your left leg along for the ride, until you complete a full set of 10 repetitions; then switch legs, and repeat with your left leg doing the work.

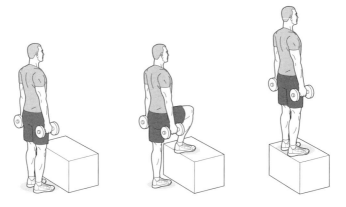

## 3 STABILITY BALL ROLLOUT
**Strengthens the rotator cuffs, scapular stabilizers, and abdominals and corrects imbalances in the shoulder girdle and trunk**

Kneel on the floor facing the ball, lean forward slightly, and place your forearms on top of the ball. Pull your belly button toward your spine. Slowly roll the ball forward by extending your forearms out in front of you and allowing your body to tilt toward the floor. Concentrate on

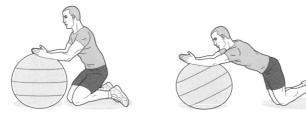

maintaining perfect alignment of your spine. Stop just before you're forced to arch your back. Hold this position for 3 seconds, and then return to the starting position, exhaling as you do so. Do up to 12 repetitions.

## 4 CABLE FACE PULL
Strengthens upper-back muscles as well as the elbow flexors and grip and helps to prevent shoulder problems

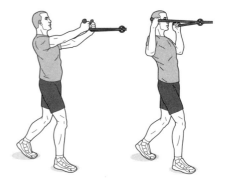

Set up a pulley with the rope attachment just above forehead level. Stand facing the pulley in a split stance, and grasp the two ends of the rope with your palms facing each other. Extend your arms straight out in front of you with the hands slightly above shoulder height. Pull the center of the rope attachment toward your forehead by retracting your shoulder blades and forcing your elbows out (not down). As the rope approaches your face, your shoulder blades should be pulled back and down, with the chest high and your hands coming even with your ears. You should feel the resistance in your midback and in the back of your shoulders. Do 10 to 12 repetitions.

## 5 SIDE STEP-UP
Strengthens the quadriceps and hips for more stable and efficient leg action

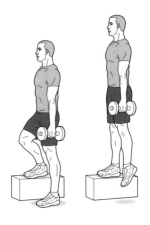

Stand with your right side facing an exercise bench or step while holding a dumbbell in your left hand with your left arm relaxed at your side. Draw your belly button gently inward toward your spine to brace your core. Place your right foot on the step, and then straighten your right leg completely so that you're now standing on the step with your left leg unsupported. Be sure not to push off the floor with your left ankle—make your right leg do all the work of lifting your body to the height of the bench. Now step back down. After completing a full set of 10 repetitions, reverse your position, and repeat with your left leg doing the work.

# STRENGTH EXERCISES FOR CYCLISTS

### 1 ELEVATED REVERSE LUNGE
**Strengthens the quadriceps for a more powerful pedal stroke**

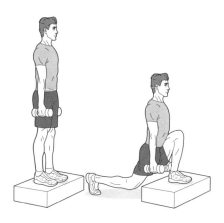

Stand on a 4- to 6-inch step with your arms resting at your sides and a dumbbell in each hand. Take a big step backward with one leg, and bend both knees until the back foot hits the ground and the back knee almost grazes the floor. Then thrust powerfully upward and forward off the back foot to return to the starting position. Be sure to maintain an upright torso posture throughout the movement. Complete 10 repetitions with one leg, rest, and then work the opposite leg.

### 2 BARBELL SQUAT
**Strengthens the gluteals, hamstrings, and quads for a more powerful pedal stroke**

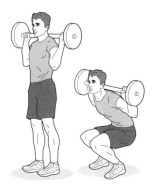

Stand with your feet slightly more than shoulder-width apart. Begin with a weighted barbell resting against your upper back and your hands grasping the bar on either side halfway between your neck and the weight plates. Draw your navel toward your spine; then lower your buttocks toward the floor as though sitting in a chair. Stop when your thighs are almost parallel to the floor; then return to the starting position. Complete 10 repetitions.

# 3 STANDING TRUNK EXTENSION
## Strengthens the lower back to reduce the risk of low-back pain resulting from cycling

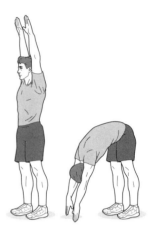

Stand tall with your feet placed slightly farther than shoulder-width apart and your arms extended straight upward, palms facing forward, with a light dumbbell (optional) in each hand. Tighten your core. Bend forward at the waist (avoid rounding your back), and reach the dumbbells toward your toes, going as far as you can without bending at the knees. Try to keep your arms more or less in line with your torso all the way down. Now return slowly to the upright position, standing tall with arms overhead. Again, maintain a neutral spine. Repeat to the point of moderate fatigue or up to 20 repetitions.

*Note:* Do not perform this exercise if you have a history of low-back injury, or if you have any reason to believe you might be prone to low-back pain.

# 4 BENT-OVER CABLE LATERAL SHOULDER EXTENSION
## Strengthens the upper back and rear shoulders to correct the forward rounding of the shoulders that often develops in cyclists

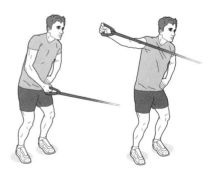

Stand in a wide stance with your knees slightly bent and your left side facing a cable pulley station with a D-handle connected to the low attachment point. Grasp the handle in your right hand using an underhand grip. Bend forward 45 degrees from the hips. Begin with your right arm extended and the handle positioned directly underneath your breastbone. Tighten your core. Now pull the handle outward and upward until your right arm is fully extended and parallel to the floor. Pause briefly and return to the starting position. Complete 10 to 12 repetitions; then reverse your position, and work the left shoulder.

## 5 GLUTEAL-HAMSTRING RAISE
**Strengthens the gluteals and hamstrings to generate more power during the pull phase of a pedal stroke**

Lie face down on the floor, and have a partner press your lower legs down into the floor just so that your body can only move from the knees up. With your arms in standard push-up position, give a slight push off the floor while you contract your hamstrings and lift your body (from knees to head) upward until you are in a fully upright kneeling position. Try to keep your torso erect throughout the movement, and use the hamstrings to pull your body up and the gluteals to finish the movement by tilting the pelvis back (just think of popping the hips forward to get your body upright). Lower yourself back to the floor. Do 8 to 10 repetitions.

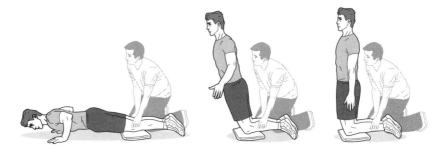

# STRENGTH EXERCISES FOR ROWERS

## 1 CABLE PULL-THROUGH
**Targets the posterior chain (hamstrings, gluteals, low back) for efficient transfer of force from legs to upper body in rowing**

Stand facing away from a cable column with the rope attachment set in the bottom position. Set your feet slightly farther than shoulder-width apart so that you have room to reach between your legs with both arms fully extended, and grasp the two ends of the rope with your palms facing each other. Bend your knees slightly, and bend forward slightly at the hips to

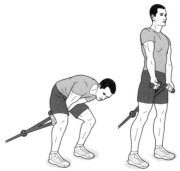

counterbalance the pull of the rope, keeping your weight on your heels. To initiate the movement, let the weight pull your hips back as if someone had a rope around your waist pulling you backward. Now begin tilting your torso forward from the hips (not the waist), and allow the weight to pull your extended arms between your legs. Avoid rounding your back. The lowering phase ends when the torso is just short of parallel with the floor, at which point you'll push through the heels and use your posterior chain to pull the rope forward between your legs and straighten your body back to the starting position. Push your hips forward, and squeeze your gluteals to lock out. Stand upright; don't lean back! Do 8 to 10 repetitions.

## 2 OVERHEAD SQUAT
**Strengthens the gluteals, hamstrings, quadriceps, core, and upper back for more powerful leg action**

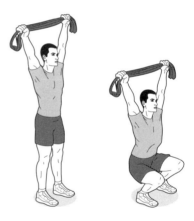

Stand with your feet slightly wider than shoulder-width apart, toes turned out slightly. Grab a rolled-up towel with an overhand grip, hands shoulder-width apart, and raise it overhead so that your shoulders are roughly in line with your heels. Squat down as far as you can without feeling discomfort in your knees or hamstrings. Return to standing to complete one full rep. Do 10 to 15 repetitions.

## 3 CABLE FRONT SHOULDER RAISE
**Strengthens the front shoulder muscles to prevent shoulder-muscle strength imbalances**

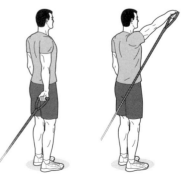

Stand facing away from a door gym or cable pulley station. Connect a handle to the low attachment point, and grasp it in your right hand with your right arm relaxed at your side, palm facing the door or cable pulley station. Set your core. Contract the muscles on the front of your shoulder, and lift the handle forward and upward, going just past the point where your arm is parallel to the floor. Pause briefly and return to the starting position. After completing a full set of 10 to 12 repetitions, work the left shoulder.

## 4 STRAIGHT-ARM LAT PULL-DOWN
### Strengthens the lower trapezius for healthy shoulders

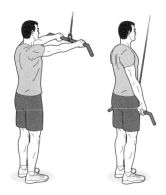

Stand facing a cable column or pull-down machine with a straight-bar attachment. Grasp the bar with a pronated (palms-down) grip and your arms extended straight in front of you with the bar at shoulder height. Keeping your torso upright and initiating the movement with your shoulder blades and upper arms, pull the bar down until it touches your upper thighs while keeping the wrists and elbows straight. When this exercise is performed correctly, you'll feel it in your midback, right at the base of your shoulder blades. Complete 8 to 10 repetitions.

## 5 L-OVER
### Strengthens the deep abdominal and oblique muscles

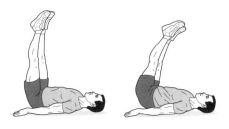

Lie face up with your arms resting at your sides and your palms flat on the floor. Extend your legs directly toward the ceiling, touch your feet together, and point your toes. Set your core. Keeping your big toes side by side, tip your legs 12 to 18 inches to the right by twisting at the hip so that your right gluteal comes off the floor. Fight the pull of gravity by maintaining stability with your abdominals and obliques. Pause for a moment, and then return slowly to the starting position, again using your core muscles to control the movement. Repeat on the left side, and continue alternating from right to left until you have completed a full set of 8–10 repetitions in each direction.

# STRENGTH EXERCISES FOR RUNNERS

## 1 SPLIT SQUAT JUMP
**Increases stride power by simulating the stride action with exaggerated upward thrust**

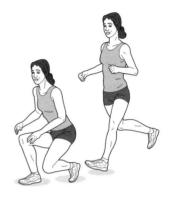

Start in a split stance with your right foot flat on the ground and your left leg slightly bent, with only the left forefoot touching the ground a half step behind the right. Lower yourself down into a deep squat, and then leap upward as high as possible. In midair, reverse the position of your legs. When you land, sink down immediately into another squat and then leap again. Use your arms to maintain balance and to generate extra upward thrust with each leap. Complete 10 to 20 jumps in each stance.

## 2 X-BAND WALK
**Strengthens the hip abductors to increase the stability of the hips and pelvis during running**

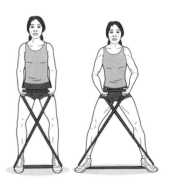

Loop a half-inch or one-inch exercise band under both feet, and stand on top of it. Your feet should be roughly 12 inches apart at the start. Cross the ends of the band to form an X, and grasp one end in each hand. Pull your chest up and shoulders back, and keep tension on the band throughout. Start walking sideways with small lateral steps. The leg that's on the side of the direction you're moving will have to overcome the band's tension to take each step. Make sure that you keep the hips and shoulders level, and don't deviate forward or backward as you step to the side. When this exercise is performed correctly, you'll feel the movement in your gluteals. Complete 10 steps in one direction, then 10 more while moving in the opposite direction.

# 3 SPLIT-STANCE DUMBBELL DEADLIFT
### Strengthens the gluteals, hips, hamstrings, quadriceps, low back, and upper back

Stand with your left foot directly beneath your left hip and your right foot half a step behind the right hip with only the toe touching the floor. Put all your weight on your left foot; use the right for balance only. Begin with dumbbells positioned on the floor directly underneath your hands as your arms hang at your sides. Bend down and grab the dumbbells. Press your left foot into the floor and stand fully upright. Concentrate on extending your left knee and hip first and then lifting your torso. Keep your weight fully on your left foot throughout this movement. Pause briefly in a standing position and then lower the dumbbells back to the floor. Complete a full set of 8 to 10, then reverse your position and do another set.

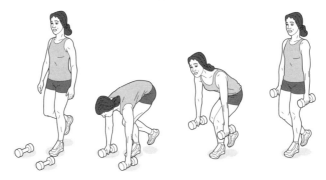

# 4 VMO DIP
### Strengthens the vastus medialis to improve the stability of the knee during running

Stand on an exercise step that's 8 to 12 inches high. Pick up your left foot, and slowly reach it toward the floor in front of the step by bending your right knee. Allow your left heel to touch the floor, but don't put any weight on it. Return to the starting position. Complete 8 to 12 repetitions; then switch legs.

*Note:* The vastus medialis is the quadriceps muscle terminating in a small bulge just above the medial side of the kneecap.

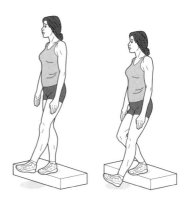

## 5 SUITCASE DEADLIFT
**Enhances the ability to resist medial tilting of the body (a cause of joint instability and overuse injuries) during the stance phase**

Stand with your arms hanging at your sides and a dumbbell in one hand. Push your hips back, bend the knees, and reach the dumbbell down as close to the floor as you can without rounding your lower back. Now stand up again. Don't allow your torso to tilt to either side while performing this movement. Complete 10 repetitions, rest for 30 seconds, and then repeat the exercise while holding the dumbbell in the opposite hand.

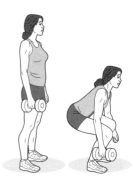

# STRENGTH EXERCISES FOR SWIMMERS

## 1 CABLE HIGH-LOW PULL
**Creates a more powerful freestyle pull by simulating the pull action under load, strengthening the upper and midback muscles**

Stand with your left side facing a cable pulley station with a D-handle attached at shoulder-to-head height. Bend your knees, and place your feet slightly more than shoulder-width apart. Use both hands to grab the handle. Your arms should be almost fully extended with your trunk twisted to the left. Now pull the handle from this position across your body and toward the floor, stopping when your hands are outside your right ankle. This is a compound movement

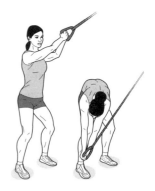

that involves twisting your torso to the right, shifting your weight from your left foot to your right foot, bending toward the floor, and using your shoulders to pull the handle across your body. Concentrate on initiating the movement with your trunk muscles. At the bottom of the movement, pause briefly, and then smoothly return to the starting position. Complete 10 repetitions. Reverse your position, and repeat the exercise.

## 2 CABLE LOW-HIGH PULL
**Strengthens the muscles responsible for body rotation during freestyle swimming for a more efficient stroke**

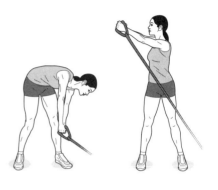

Connect a D-handle to a cable pulley station at ankle height. Stand in a wide stance with your left side facing the cable pulley station and most of your weight on the left foot. Grasp the handle in both hands, beginning with the handle just outside your lower left shin. Using both arms, pull the cable upward and across your body, keeping your arms straight and finishing with your hands above your right shoulder. Avoid rounding your back. Return smoothly to the starting position. Complete 10 repetitions. Reverse your position, and repeat the exercise.

## 3 PUSH-UP AND REACH
**Strengthens the chest, triceps, and shoulder stabilizers for greater shoulder stability and lower risk of "swimmer's shoulder"**

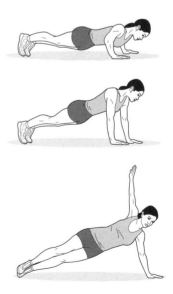

Begin by doing a standard push-up. At the top of the movement, when your arms are completely straight, twist your body to the right and reach straight toward the ceiling with your right arm. Follow the movement of your hand with your eyes. Pause for 1 second, and then put that hand back down and twist left, reaching up with your left hand. One push-up with reaches to both sides counts as 1 repetition. Do 10 to 15 repetitions. If you can't do at least 10 regular push-ups, do half push-ups (where you lower your chest only halfway to the floor).

# 4 CABLE EXTERNAL SHOULDER ROTATION
### Strengthens the rotator cuff muscles and reduces risk of injury

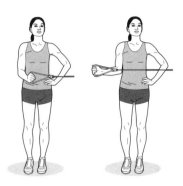

Stand with your left side facing a cable pulley station. Grasp the D-handle in your right hand, and begin with your right arm bent 90 degrees so that your forearm is pointing toward the cable pulley station across your belly. Now rotate your shoulder externally, and pull the handle across your body, keeping your elbow and upper arm pressed against your right side. Return to the starting position. Complete 10 repetitions; then repeat with your left arm.

# 5 ONE-ARM DUMBBELL SNATCH
### Attenuates muscle imbalances created by swimming by essentially reversing the freestyle arm-pull action

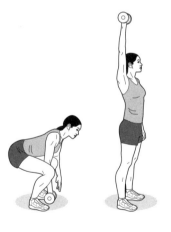

Assume a wide stance with a single dumbbell placed on the floor between your feet. Bend your knees, tilt forward from the hips, and grasp the dumbbell with your right hand using an overhand grip (knuckles facing forward). Begin with your right arm fully extended. The objective of this exercise is to lift the dumbbell in a straight line from the floor to a point directly overhead. To do this, begin by contracting your gluteals, hamstrings, and lower back so that the dumbbell rises to thigh height as you assume an upright standing position. From this point, keep the dumbbell moving in a straight line close to your body by bending your elbow and pulling from the shoulder. As the dumbbell approaches head level, rotate and extend your arm until it is pointing toward the ceiling. Pause briefly, and then reverse the movement, allowing the dumbbell to come to rest again on the floor briefly before you initiate the next lift. Complete 10 to 12 repetitions; then switch to the right arm.

# STRENGTH EXERCISES FOR TRIATHLETES

### 1 ELEVATED REVERSE LUNGE
**Strengthens the quadriceps for a more powerful pedal stroke**

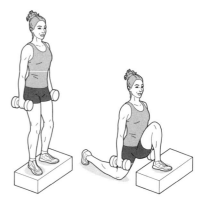

Stand on a 4- to 6-inch step with your arms resting at your sides and a dumbbell in each hand. Take a big step backward with one leg, and bend both knees until the back foot hits the ground and the back knee almost grazes the floor. Then thrust powerfully upward and forward off the back foot to return to the starting position. Be sure to maintain an upright torso posture throughout the movement. Complete 10 repetitions with one leg, rest, and then work the opposite leg.

### 2 ONE-LEG SQUAT
**Trains the hip abductors and external rotators to maintain hip stability during a single-leg movement similar to running**

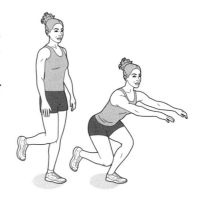

Stand on your right foot, and bend the left leg slightly to elevate the left foot a few inches above the floor. Lower your buttocks slowly toward the floor, keeping most of your weight on the heel of your support foot. Reach the left leg either behind your body (easier) or in front of your body (harder) to keep it out of the way and to help maintain balance. Squat as low as you can go without your buttocks swinging outward (a sign that the targeted muscles have become overwhelmed and that other muscles have been activated to take up the slack). Return to the starting position. Do 8 to 10 squats on each foot.

## 3 SUITCASE DEADLIFT
Enhances the ability to resist medial tilting of the body (a major cause of joint instability and overuse injuries) during the stance phase of running

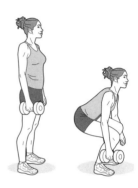

Stand with your arms hanging at your sides and a dumbbell in one hand. Push your hips back, bend the knees, and reach the dumbbell down as close to the floor as you can without rounding your lower back. Now stand up again. Don't allow your torso to tilt to either side while performing this movement. Complete 10 repetitions, rest for 30 seconds, and then repeat the exercise while holding the dumbbell in the opposite hand.

## 4 PUSH-UP AND REACH
Strengthens the chest, triceps, and shoulder stabilizers for greater shoulder stability and reduced risk of "swimmer's shoulder"

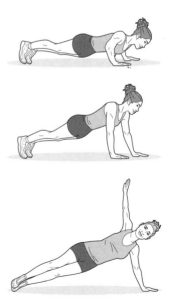

Begin by doing a standard push-up. At the top of the movement, when your arms are completely straight, twist your body to the right and reach straight toward the ceiling with your right arm. Follow the movement of your hand with your eyes. Pause for 1 second, and then put that hand back down and twist left, reaching up with your left hand. One push-up with reaches to both sides counts as 1 repetition. Do 10 to 15 repetitions. If you can't do at least 10 regular push-ups, do half push-ups (where you lower your chest only halfway to the floor).

# 5 ONE-ARM DUMBBELL SNATCH
## Attenuates muscle imbalances created by swimming by essentially reversing the freestyle arm-pull action

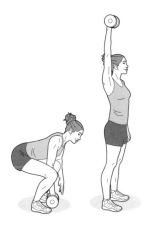

Assume a wide stance with a single dumbbell placed on the floor between your feet. Bend your knees, tilt forward from the hips, and grasp the dumbbell with your right hand using an overhand grip (knuckles facing forward). Begin with your right arm fully extended. The objective of this exercise is to lift the dumbbell in a straight line from the floor to a point directly overhead. To do this, begin by contracting your gluteals, hamstrings, and lower back so that the dumbbell rises to thigh height as you assume an upright standing position. From this point, keep the dumbbell moving in a straight line close to your body by bending your elbow and pulling from the shoulder. As the dumbbell approaches head level, rotate and extend your arm until it is pointing toward the ceiling. Pause briefly, and then reverse the movement, allowing the dumbbell to come to rest again on the floor briefly before you initiate the next lift. Complete 10 to 12 repetitions; then switch to the right arm.

# REFERENCES

Achten, J., S. L. Halson, L. Moseley, M. P. Rayson, A. Casey, and A. E. Jeukendrup. 2004. Higher Dietary Carbohydrate Content During Intensified Running Training Results in Better Maintenance of Performance and Mood State. *Journal of Applied Physiology* 96: 1331–40.

Aoi, W., H. Yamauchi, M. Iwasa, K. Mune, K. Furuta, W. Tanimura, S. Wada, and A. Higashi. 2012, August 20. Combined Light Exercise After Meal Intake Suppresses Postprandial Serum Triglyceride. *Medicine and Science in Sports and Exercise.*

Bakshi, R., Y. Bhambhani, and H. Madill. 1991. The Effects of Task Preference on Performance During Purposeful and Non-purposeful Activities. *American Journal of Occupational Therapy* 45(10): 912–16.

Bale, P., D. Bradbury, and E. Colley. 1986. Anthropometric and Training Variables Related to 10 km Running Performance. *British Journal of Sports Medicine* 20(4): 170–73.

Ball, M. F., L. H. Kyle, and J. J. Canary. 1967. Comparative Effects of Caloric Restriction and Metabolic Acceleration on Body Composition in Obesity. *Journal of Clinical Endocrinology and Metabolism* 27(2): 273.

Beis, L. Y., L. Willkomm, R. Ross, Z. Bekele, B. Wolde, B. Fudge, and Y. P. Pitsiladis. 2011. Food and Macronutrient Intake of Elite Ethiopian Distance Runners. *Journal of the International Society of Sports Nutrition* 19(8): 7.

Berardi, J. M., T. B. Price, E. E. Noreen, and P. W. Lemon. 2006. Postexercise Muscle Glycogen Recovery Enhanced with a Carbohydrate-Protein Supplement. *Medicine and Science in Sports and Exercise* 38(6): 1106–13.

Bes-Rastrollo, M., N. M. Wedick, M. A. Martinez-Gonzalez, T. Y. Li, L. Sampson, and F. B. Hu. 2009. Prospective Study of Nut Consumption, Long-Term Weight Change, and Obesity Risk in Women. *American Journal of Clinical Nutrition* 89(6): 1913–19.

Billat, V. L., A. Demarle, J. Slawinski, M. Paiva, and J. P. Koralsztein. 2001. Physical and Training Characteristics of Top-Class Marathon Runners. *Medicine and Science in Sports and Exercise* 33(12): 2089–97.

Boyles, S. 2012, February 20. Gluten Sensitivity: Fact or Fad? Analysis Questions Benefits of Gluten-Free Diet for Many. WebMD. http://www.webmd.com/diet/news/20120220/gluten-sensitivity-fact-or-fad.

Butryn, M. L., S. Phelan, J. O. Hill, and R. R. Wing. 2007. Consistent Self-Monitoring of Weight: A Key Component of Successful Weight Loss Maintenance. *Obesity* 15(12): 3091–96.

Cermak, N. M., M. J. Gibala, and L. J. van Loon. 2012. Nitrate Supplementation's Improvement of 10-km Time-Trial Performance in Trained Cyclists. *International Journal of Sports Nutrition and Exercise Metabolism* 22(1): 64–71.

Ciampolini, M., D. Lovell-Smith, and M. Sifone. 2010. Sustained Self-Regulation of Energy Intake: Loss of Weight in Overweight Subjects, Maintenance of Weight in Normal-Weight Subjects. *Nutrition and Metabolism* 7(4).

Ciccolo, J. T., J. B. Bartholomew, M. Stults-Kolehmainen, J. Seifert, and R. Portman. 2009. Relationship Between Body Weight and Health-Related Quality of Life Amongst a Large Group of Highly Active Individuals. Paper presented at the Society for Behavioral Medicine, Montreal, Canada.

Creer, A. R., M. D. Ricard, R. K. Conlee, G. L. Hoyt, and A. C. Parcell. 2004. Neural, Metabolic, and Performance Adaptations to Four Weeks of High Intensity Sprint-Interval Training in Trained Cyclists. *International Journal of Sports Medicine* 25(2): 92–98.

Cureton, K. J., and P. B. Sparling. 1980. Distance Running, Performance, and Metabolic Responses to Running in Men and Women with Excess Weight Experimentally Equated. *Medicine and Science in Sports and Exercise* 12(4): 288–94.

Dansinger, M. L., J. A. Gleason, J. L. Griffith, H. P. Selker, and E. J. Schaefer. 2005. Comparison of the Atkins, Ornish, Weight Watchers, and Zone Diet for Weight Loss and Heart Disease Risk Reduction: A Randomized Trial. *JAMA* 293(1): 43–53.

Davis, J. M., S. Sadri, R. G. Sargent, and D. Ward. 1989. Weight Control and Calorie Expenditure: Thermogenic Effect of Pre-prandial and Post-prandial Exercise. *Addictive Behaviors* 14(3): 347–51.

De Castro, J. M. 2007. The Time of Day and the Proportions of Macronutrients Eaten Are Related to Total Daily Food Intake. *British Journal of Nutrition* 98(5): 1077–83.

Dennis, E. A., A. L. Dengo, D. L. Comber, K. D. Flack, J. Savia, K. P. Davy, and B. M. Davy. 2010. Water Consumption Increases Weight Loss During a Hypocaloric Diet Intervention in Middle-Aged and Older Adults. *Obesity* 18(2): 300–7.

Deutz, R. C., D. Benardot, D. E. Martin, and M. M. Cody. 2000. Relationship Between Energy Deficits and Body Composition in Elite Female Gymnasts and Runners. *Medicine and Science in Sports and Exercise* 32(3): 659–68.

Dumke, C. L., C. M. Pfaffenroth, J. M. McBride, and G. O. McCauley. 2010. Relationship Between Muscle Strength, Power, and Stiffness and Running Economy in Trained Male Runners. *International Journal of Sports Physiology and Performance* 5(2): 249–61.

Farshchi, H. R., M. A. Taylor, and I. A. Macdonald. 2004a. Decreased Thermic Effect of Food After an Irregular Compared with a Regular Meal Pattern in Healthy Lean Women. *International Journal of Obesity-Related Metabolic Disorders* 28(5): 653–60.

Farshchi, H. R., M. A. Taylor, and I. A. Macdonald. 2004b. Regular Meal Frequency Creates More Appropriate Insulin Sensitivity and Lipid Profiles Compared with Irregular Meal Frequency in Healthy Lean Women. *European Journal of Clinical Nutrition* 58(7): 1071–77.

Fisher, J. O., B. J. Rolls, and L. L. Birch. 2003. Children's Bite Size and Intake of an Entrée Are Greater with Large Portions Than with Age-Appropriate or Self-Selected Portions. *American Journal of Clinical Nutrition* 77: 1164–70.

Fiskerstrand, A., and K. S. Seiler. 2004. Training and Performance Characteristics Among Norwegian International Rowers, 1970–2001. *Scandinavian Journal of Medicine and Science in Sports* 14: 303–10.

Fleming, J., M. J. Sharman, N. G. Avery, D. M. Love, A. L. Gómez, T. P. Scheet, W. J. Kraemer, and J. S. Volek. 2003. Endurance Capacity and High-Intensity Exercise Performance Responses to a High-Fat Diet. *International Journal of Sport Nutrition and Exercise Metabolism* 13(4): 466–78.

Flood, J. E., and B. J. Rolls. 2007. Soup Preloads in a Variety of Forms Reduce Meal Energy Intake. *Appetite* 49(3): 626–34.

Framson, C., A. R. Kristal, J. M. Shenk, A. J. Littman, S. Zeliadt, and D. Benitez. 2009. Development and Validation of the Mindful Eating Questionnaire. *Journal of the American Dietetic Association* 109(8): 1439–44.

Fudge, B. W., C. Easton, D. Kingsmore, F. K. Kiplamai, V. O. Onywera, K. R. Westerterp, B. Kayser, T. D. Noakes, and Y. P. Pitsiladis. 2008. Elite Kenyan Endurance Runners Are Hydrated Day-to-Day with ad Libitum Fluid Intake. *Medicine and Science in Sports and Exercise* 40(6): 1171–79.

Fudge, B. W., K. R. Westerterp, F. K. Kiplamai, V. O. Onywera, M. K. Boit, B. Kayser, and Y. P. Pitsiladis. 2006. Evidence of Negative Energy Balance Using Doubly Labeled Water in Elite Kenyan Endurance Runners Prior to Competition. *British Journal of Nutrition* 95(1): 59–66.

Fuhrman, J., B. Sarter, D. Glaser, and S. Acocella. 2010. Changing Perceptions of Hunger on a High Nutrient Density Diet. *Nutrition Journal* 9: 51.

Gerlach, K. E., H. W. Burton, J. M. Dorn, J. J. Leddy, and P. J. Horvath. 2008. Fat Intake and Injury in Female Runners. *Journal of the International Society of Sports Nutrition* 5(1). http://www.ncbi.nlm.nih.gov/pubmed/18173851.

Giovannini, M., E. Verduci, S. Scaglioni, E. Salvatici, M. Bonza, E. Riva, and C. Agostoni. 2008. Breakfast: A Good Habit, Not a Repetitive Custom. *Journal of International Medical Research* 36(4): 613–24.

Good, C. K., N. Holschuh, A. M. Albertson, and A. L. Eldridge. 2008. Whole Grain Consumption and Body Mass Index in Adult Women: An Analysis of NHANES 1999–2000 and the USDA Pyramid Servings Database. *Journal of the American College of Nutrition* 27(1): 80–87.

Goodman-Larson, A., K. Johnson, and K. Shevlin. 2003. The Effect of Meal Frequency on Preprandial Resting Metabolic Rate. *University of Wisconsin–La Crosse Journal of Undergraduate Research* 6: 1–4.

Haupt, A. 2011, July 20. Health Buzz: Restaurant Calorie Counts Often Inaccurate. *U.S. News and World Report.*

Havenar, J. M., and M. Lochbaum. 2007. Differences in Participation Motives of First-Time Marathon Finishers and Pre-race Dropouts. *Journal of Sport Behavior* 30(3): 270–79.

Hecht, S., D. Vigil, J. Luftman, A. Vasco, I. Gardner, L. Huston, and R. Contreras. 2007. Body Composition Analysis and Performance in Triathletes. Paper presented at the Annual Meeting of the American Medical Society for Sports Medicine, Albuquerque, New Mexico.

Hill, A. M., J. D. Buckley, K. J. Murphy, and P. R. Howe. 2007. Combining Fish-Oil Supplements with Regular Aerobic Exercise Improves Body Composition and Cardiovascular Disease Risk Factors. *American Journal of Clinical Nutrition* 85(5): 1267–74.

Hollis, J. F., C. M. Gullion, V. J. Stevens, P. J. Brantley, L. J. Appel, J. D. Ard, C. M. Champagne, A. Dalcin, T. P. Erlinger, K. Funk, D. Laferriere, P. H. Lin, C. M. Loria, C. Samuel-Hodge, W. M. Vollmer, and L. P. Svetkey. 2008. Weight Loss During the Intensive Intervention Phase of the Weight-Loss Maintenance Trial. *American Journal of Preventive Medicine* 35(2): 118–26.

Hsu, F. C., L. Lenchik, B. J. Nicklas, K. Lohman, T. C. Register, J. Mychaleckyj, C. D. Langefeld, B. I. Freedman, D. W. Bowden, and J. J. Carr. 2005. Heritability of Body Composition Measured by DXA in the Diabetes Heart Study. *Obesity Research* 13(2): 312–19.

Jarvis, M., L. McNaughton, S. Seddon, and D. Thompson. 2002. The Acute 1-Week Effects of the Zone Diet on Body Composition, Blood Lipid Levels, and Performance in Recreational Endurance Athletes. *Journal of Strength and Conditioning Research* 16(1): 50–57.

Knechtle, B., A. Wirth, C. Alexander Rüst, and T. Rosemann. 2011. The Relationship Between Anthropometry and Split Performance in Recreational Male Ironman Triathletes. *Asian Journal of Sports Medicine* 2(1): 23–30.

Leidy, H. J., and W. W. Campbell. 2011. The Effect of Eating Frequency on Appetite Control and Food Intake: Brief Synopsis of Controlled Feeding Studies. *Journal of Nutrition* 141(1): 154–57.

LeSauter, J., N. Hoque, M. Weintraub, D. W. Pfaff, and R. Silver. 2009. Stomach Ghrelin-Secreting Cells as Food-Entrainable Circadian Clocks. *Proceedings of the National Academy of Sciences* 106(32): 13582–87.

Lewis, B. A., B. H. Marcus, R. R. Pate, and A. L. Dunn. 2002. Psychosocial Mediators of Physical Activity Behavior Among Adults and Children. *American Journal of Preventive Medicine* 23 (2 Supplement): 26–35.

Lunn, W. R., J. A. Finn, and R. S. Axtell. 2009. Effects of Sprint Interval Training and Body Weight Reduction on Power to Weight Ratio in Experienced Cyclists. *Journal of Strength and Conditioning Research* 23(4): 1217–24.

Macdermid, P. W., and S. R. Stannard. 2006. A Whey-Supplemented, High-Protein Diet Versus a High-Carbohydrate Diet: Effects on Endurance Cycling Performance. *International Journal of Sports Nutrition and Exercise Metabolism* 16(1): 65–77.

Martinez-Lagunas, V., Z. Ding, J. R. Bernard, B. Wang, and J. L. Ivy. 2010. Added Protein Maintains Efficacy of a Low-Carbohydrate Sports Drink. *Journal of Strength and Conditioning Research* 24(1): 48–59.

Martins, C., L. M. Morgan, S. R. Bloom, and M. D. Robertson. 2007. Effect of Exercise on Gut Peptides, Energy Intake, and Appetite. *Journal of Endocrinology* 193(2): 251–58.

McArdle, W. D., F. I. Katch, and V. L. Katch. 2005. *Sports and Exercise Nutrition.* Philadelphia, Pa.: Lippincott, Williams & Wilkins.

McClernon, F. J., W. S. Yancy Jr., J. A. Eberstein, R. C. Atkins, and E. C. Westman. 2007. The Effects of a Low-Carbohydrate Ketogenic Diet and a Low-Fat Diet on Mood, Hunger, and Other Self-Reported Symptoms. *Obesity* 15(1): 182–87.

Meinz, D. "Fad Diets Versus Dietary Guidelines." http://www.davidmeinz.com/diets/index.html.

Melby, C. L., K. L. Osterberg, A. Resch, B. Davy, S. Johnson, and K. Davy. 2002. Effect of Carbohydrate Ingestion During Exercise on Post-Exercise Substrate Oxidation and Energy Intake. *International Journal of Sport Nutrition and Exercise Metabolism* 12(3): 294–309.

Micha, R., S. K. Wallace, and D. Mozzafarian. 2010. Red and Processed Meat Consumption and Risk of Incident Coronary Heart Disease, Stroke, and Diabetes Mellitus: A Systematic Review and Meta-analysis. *Circulation* 121: 2271–83.

Michels, K. B., and A. A. Wolk. 2002. A Prospective Study of Variety of Healthy Foods and Mortality in Women. *International Journal of Epidemiology* 31: 847–54.

Monteleone, P., F. Piscitelli, P. Scognamiglio, A. M. Monteleone, B. Canestrelli, V. Di Marzo, and M. Maj. 2012. Hedonic Eating Is Associated with Increased Peripheral Levels of Ghrelin and the Endocannabinoid 2-Arachidonoyl-Glycerol in Healthy Humans: A Pilot Study. *Journal of Clinical Endocrinology and Metabolism* 97(6): E917–24.

Mozaffarian, D., T. Hao, E. B. Rimm, W. C. Willett, and F. B. Hu. 2011. Changes in Diet and Lifestyle and Long-Term Weight Gain in Women and Men. *New England Journal of Medicine* 364: 2392–2404.

Mujika, I., J. C. Chatard, T. Busso, A. Geyssant, F. Barale, and L. Lacoste. 1995. Effects of Training on Performance in Competitive Swimming. *Canadian Journal of Applied Physiology* 20: 395–406.

Mustelin, L., K. H. Pietiläinen, A. Rissanen, A. R. Sovijärvi, P. Piirilä, J. Naukkarinen, L. Peltonen, J. Kaprio, and H. Yki-Järvinen. 2008. Acquired Obesity and Poor Physical Fitness Impair Expression of Genes of Mitochondrial Oxidative Phosphorylation in Monozygotic Twins Discordant for Obesity. *American Journal of Physiology, Endocrinology, and Metabolism* 295(1): E148–54.

Neal, C. M., A. M. Hunter, and S. D. Galloway. 2011. A 6-Month Analysis of Training-Intensity Distribution and Physiological Adaptation in Ironman Triathletes. *Journal of Sports Science* 29(14): 1515–23.

Newby, P. K., F. B. Hu, E. B. Rimm, S. A. Smith-Warner, D. Feskanich, L. Sampson, and W. C. Willett. 2003. Reproducibility and Validity of the Diet Quality Index Revised as Assessed by Use of a Food-Frequency Questionnaire. *American Journal of Clinical Nutrition* 78(5): 941–49.

Nieman, D. C., N. D. Gillitt, D. A. Henson, W. Sha, R. A. Shanely, A. M. Knab, L. Cialdella-Kam, and F. Jin. 2012. Bananas as an Energy Source During Exercise: A Metabolomics Approach. *PLoS One* 7(5). http://www.ncbi.nlm.nih.gov/pubmed/22616015.

Onywera, V. O., F. K. Kiplamai, M. K. Boit, and Y. P. Pitsiladis. 2004. Food and Macronutrient Intake of Elite Kenyan Distance Runners. *International Journal of Sport Nutrition and Exercise Metabolism* 14(6): 709–19.

Padilla, S., I. Mujika, G. Cuesta, and J. J. Goiriena. 1999. Level Ground and Uphill Cycling Ability in Professional Road Cycling. *Medicine and Science in Sports and Exercise* 31(6): 878–85.

Painter, J. E., B. Wansink, and J. B. Hieggelke. 2002. How Visibility and Convenience Influence Candy Consumption. *Appetite* 38(3): 237–38.

Parker-Pope, T. 2011, January 7. Nutrition Advice from the China Study. Well blog. *New York Times.* http://well.blogs.nytimes.com/2011/01/07/nutrition-advice-from-the-china-study/.

Paton, C. D., and W. G. Hopkins. 2005. Combining Explosive and High-Resistance Training Improves Performance in Competitive Cyclists. *Journal of Strength and Conditioning Research* 19(4): 826–30.

Peoples, G. E., P. L. McLennan, P. R. Howe, and H. Groeller. 2008. Fish Oil Reduces Heart Rate and Oxygen Consumption During Exercise. *Journal of Cardiovascular Pharmacology* 52(6): 540–47.

Popkin, B. M., and S. J. Nielsen. 2003. Patterns and Trends in Food Portion Sizes, 1977–1998. *JAMA* 289(4): 450–53.

Portman, Robert, and John Ivy. 2011. *Hardwired for Fitness: The Revolutionary Way to Lose Weight, Have More Energy, and Improve Body Composition—Naturally.* Laguna Beach, CA: Basic Health Publications.

Reel, J. J. 1997. Social Physique Anxiety and Weight Pressures Among Female College Swimmers. *Journal of Applied Sport Psychology* 9: S147.

Res, P. T., B. Groen, B. Pennings, M. Beleen, G. A. Wallis, A. P. Gijsen, J. M. Senden, and L. J. van Loon. 2012. Protein Ingestion Before Sleep Improves Postexercise Overnight Recovery. *Medicine and Science in Sports and Exercise* 44(8): 1560–69.

Rosell, M., N. N. Håkansson, and A. Wolk. 2006. Association Between Dairy Food Consumption and Weight Change over 9 y in 19,352 Perimenopausal Women. *American Journal of Clinical Nutrition* 84(6): 1481–88.

Rowell, L. B., E. J. Masoro, and M. J. Spencer. 1965. Splanchnic Metabolism in Exercising Man. *Journal of Applied Physiology* 20(5): 1032–37.

Rowlands, D. S., and W. G. Hopkins. 2002. Effects of High-Fat and High-Carbohydrate Diets on Metabolism and Performance in Cycling. *Metabolism* 51(6): 678–90.

Rubio-Tapia, A., A. F. Ludviggson, T. L. Brantner, J. A. Murray, and J. E. Everhart. 2012, July 31. The Prevalence of Celiac Disease in the United States. *American Journal of Gastroenterology.* doi: 10.1038/ajg.2012.219.

Sato, K., and M. Mokha. 2009. Does Core Strength Training Influence Running Kinetics, Lower-Extremity Stability, and 5,000-M Performance in Runners? *Journal of Strength and Conditioning Research* 23(1): 133–40.

Sherman, W. M., and G. S. Wimer. 1991. Insufficient Dietary Carbohydrate During Training: Does It Impair Athletic Performance? *International Journal of Sport Nutrition* 1(1): 28–44.

Sherman, W. M., J. A. Doyle, D. R. Lamb, and R. H. Strauss. 1993. Dietary Carbohydrate, Muscle Glycogen, and Exercise Performance During 7 Days of Training. *American Journal of Clinical Nutrition* 57(1): 27–31.

Smeets, A. J., and M. S. Westerterp-Plantenga. 2008. Acute Effect on Metabolism and Appetite Profile of One Meal Difference in the Lower Range of Meal Frequency. *British Journal of Nutrition* 99(6): 1316–21.

Stensel, D. 2010. Exercise, Appetite, and Appetite-Regulating Hormones: Implications for Food Intake and Weight Control. *Annals of Nutrition and Metabolism* 57(2): 36–42.

Støren, O., J. Helgerud, E. M. Støa, and J. Hoff. 2008. Maximal Strength Training Improves Running Economy in Distance Runners. *Medicine and Science in Sports and Exercise* 40(6): 1087–92.

Stroebele, N., and J. M. Castro. 2004. Television Viewing Is Associated with an Increase in Meal Frequency in Humans. *Appetite* 42(1): 111–13.

Stults-Kolehmainen, M., J. T. Ciccolo, J. B. Bartholomew, J. Seifert, and R. Portman. 2009. Age-Related Changes in Motivation to Exercise Among Highly Active Individuals. *Annals of Behavioral Medicine* Supplement 1: D168.

Thompson, S. H. 2007. Characteristics of the Female Athlete Triad in Collegiate Cross-Country Runners. *Journal of American College Health* 56(2): 129–36.

Thomson, R., G. D. Brinkworth, J. D. Buckley, M. Noakes, and P. M. Clifton. 2007. Good Agreement Between Bioelectrical Impedance and Dual-Energy X-ray Absorptiometry for Estimating Changes in Body Composition During Weight Loss in Overweight Young Women. *Clinical Nutrition* 26(6): 771–77.

Urban, L. E., M. A. McCrory, G. E. Dallal, S. K. Das, E. Saltzman, J. L. Weber, and S. B. Roberts. 2011. Accuracy of Stated Energy Contents of Restaurant Foods. *JAMA* 306(3): 287–93.

Van Wormer, J. J., A. M. Martinez, B. C. Martinson, A. L. Crain, G. A. Benson, D. L. Cosentino, and N. P. Pronk. 2009. Self-Weighing Promotes Weight Loss for Obese Adults. *American Journal of Preventive Medicine* 36(1): 70–73.

Wansink B., C. R. Payne, and P. Chandon. 2007. Internal and External Cues of Meal Cessation: The French Paradox Redux? *Obesity* 15(12): 2920–24.

White, L. J., R. H. Dressendorfer, E. Holland, S. C. McCoy, and M. A. Ferguson. 2005. Increased Caloric Intake Soon After Exercise in Cold Water. *International Journal of Sport Nutrition and Exercise Metabolism* 15(1): 38–47.

Williams, M. B., P. B. Raven, D. L. Fogt, and J. L. Ivy. 2003. Effects of Recovery Beverages on Glycogen Restoration and Endurance Exercise Performance. *Journal of Strength and Conditioning Research* 17(1): 12–19.

Williams, P. T. 2007. Maintaining Vigorous Activity Attenuates 7-Year Weight Gain in 8,340 Runners. *Medicine and Science in Sports and Exercise* 39(5): 801–9.

Wing, R. R., and S. Phelan. 2005. Long-Term Weight Loss Maintenance. *American Journal of Clinical Nutrition* 82(1 Suppl): 222S–25S.

Young, L. R., and M. Nestle. 2007. Portion Sizes and Obesity: Responses of Fast-Food Companies. *Journal of Public Health Policy* 28(2): 238–48.

# INDEX

# ABOUT THE AUTHOR

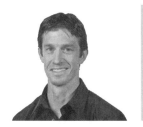

**MATT FITZGERALD** is a highly acclaimed endurance sportswriter. His awards include the 2011 min Award for Best Opinion/Commentary. In 2012 he was named a finalist for the William Hill Sports Book of the Year for *Iron War*, his account of the great triathlon rivalry between Dave Scott and Mark Allen. Matt's other books include *The New Rules of Marathon and Half Marathon Nutrition*, *Brain Training for Runners*, and *Triathlete Magazine's Essential Week-by-Week Training Guide*. His writing has also appeared in major publications including *Bicycling, Competitor, Inside Triathlon, Outside, Runner's World, Shape, Triathlete*, and *Velo*.

A certified sports nutritionist, Matt has consulted for several sports nutrition companies and conducts peer reviews for the *Journal of the International Society of Sports Nutrition*. Matt has coached runners and triathletes since 2001 and currently serves as a Training Intelligence Specialist for PEAR Sports.

An endurance athlete himself for more than 30 years, Matt now lives in northern California with his wife, Nataki.

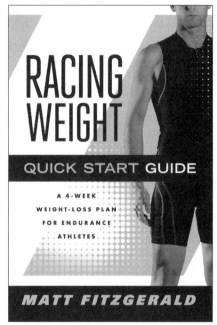
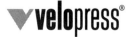